The Potent Self

A GUIDE TO SPONTANEITY

Moshe Feldenkrais

Edited by Michaeleen Kimmey

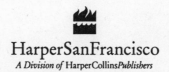

HarperSanFrancisco
A Division of HarperCollins*Publishers*

FIRST HARPERCOLLINS PAPERBACK EDITION PUBLISHED IN 1992.

Library of Congress Cataloging-in-Publication Data

Feldenkrais, Moshé.
    The potent self: a guide to spontaneity / Moshé Feldendrais :
edited by Michaeleen Kimmey. — 1st HarperCollins pbk. ed.
        p.   cm.
    Reprint. Originally published: San Francisco : Harper & Row,
c1985.
        ISBN 0-06-250324-3 (alk. paper)
        1. Feldenkrais method.   2. Spontaneity (Personality trait)
I. Kimmey, Michaeleen.   II. Title.
    [RC489.F44F444   1992]
    158'.1—dc20
                                                    91-55443
                                                    CIP

92 93 94 95 96 MCN 10 9 8 7 6 5 4 3 2 1

Contents

Editor's Note

This manuscript was written for the general reader, before, during, and after the more scientifically oriented *Body and Mature Behavior*, which was published in 1949. As a scientist, Dr. Feldenkrais was interested in what could be done to effect change and desired a friendly attitude, if not support, for his method from the scientific community at large. For this reason he chose not to publish this exhaustive analysis of the underlying emotional mechanisms that lead to widespread infantile dependency in our society.

In the intervening forty years, his method has gained a broad spectrum of acceptance in the community of scientists. It is now time to present to the public what was written for them. At the urging of family and friends he decided to publish it in the hope that it would be of some use to the present generation.

I have taken the liberty of alternating gender voice from chapter to chapter. My suggestion is that you read this aloud, as he used language as it is spoken, not as it is written.

On July 1st, 1984, at the age of 80, Moshe Feldenkrais died as peacefully as he lived. Those of us who had the good fortune to encounter this truly human spirit hope you will discover some of his great humanity in his words.

M. K.

Preface

The present is only a fleeting moment, an instant that passes at once into the past. It then escapes our influence so utterly that it is beyond the reach of the wildest imagination. Most people behave as if their future is completely and irrevocably forfeited by what they have done in the past. This conviction is so deep that they continue to live in the past while in the present and thus confirm their expectation, namely that the past is binding, and they cannot but repeat themselves over again and again.

The present is the time in which we live, and what we do with our present selves is the most important thing. For the past is carried into the future through our present selves; what we do now is the most important factor for tomorrow. If we do nothing to change our emotional pattern of behavior, tomorrow will resemble yesterday in most details except the date. The past is history, the future only a guess—this present makes them both what they are.

Do not try to forget the past; it is impossible to forget the past without forgetting oneself at the same time. You may imagine that you have forgotten one or another unwanted detail, but it is stamped in some part of your body. Yet that past experience, awful as it may have been, can be used now to make your present a vital basis for a fuller, more absorbingly interesting future. When you have learned to accept the past and you have made peace with it, then it will leave you in peace. My contention is that the maturing process should never come to a standstill in any plane of human activity if life is to be a healthy process. Maturity itself is a process, and not a final state; it is the process whereby past personal experience is broken up into its constituent parts and new patterns are formed out of them to fit the present circumstances of the environment and the present state of the body.

At first glance it may seem that undue importance is attached to the problem of sex and too much space alloted to it. The thoughtful reader will soon recognize that there is no intention to bring this problem to a position of predominance in human behavior. Although I as a teacher set out to increase the student's mature sexual potency, it is not for the sake of lust or pleasurable indulgence as found in the immature person. Sexual maturity arrives at the end of the development period, and is the most vulnerable function because of that. All the consequences of improper and inexpedient habits formed through personal experience in the preceding growth period bear on it and mark this function more than any other function that matures earlier. Any arrest in development that may occur during this susceptible period of childhood and adolescence will of necessity affect the function that has yet to mature. Similarly, it is impossible to correct and reform adequately the general use of oneself without recovering sexual spontaneity. There are many who do not consider themselves lacking in this respect but still feel that they do not live fully, that life is an empty obligation with no real interest, and that they should have given a better account of themselves—they have probably never known sexual spontaneity, and have never, although they may argue in all sincerity to the contrary, enjoyed full active potency. They vegetate on a lower level of existence, from which it is impossible to rise without learning the healthy use of self that leads to spontaneous, full, and active potency. This cannot be achieved without becoming an active and evolving person at the same time.

The healthy person has a fuller and altogether more gratifying sexual life than the compulsive person. And a healthy sex drive does not become that constant nagging feeling familiar to many, that absorbs the entire personality throughout the waking and sleeping life. The ability to spontaneously mobilize all one's abilities for the immediate task in hand is normally enjoyed by those who are also capable of full sexual gratification. The aim of this book is to give the reader the means of achieving such a satisfying self-realization that the problem of sex should recede from the central position which it now occupies to the place where it belongs—a cardinal and honorable place, in its own time, but not all the time.

Introduction: Love Thyself as Thy Neighbor

The admirable saying "Love thy neighbor as thyself" is the core of all religions. It has served humanity well and is still a goal to be treasured by all humanists. Yet there is also room for the symmetrical saying. The best intentions when enacted compulsively yield opposite results. Compulsively religious people have done enough harm in particular cases in the past, and are still doing so, to outweigh the blessings of religious ethics. Our education is permeated with the idea of loving one's neighbor as oneself, but far too often this idea is instilled with such rigor and absolutism as to stamp out all spontaneity. Many people become "good" not by learning to live in good neighborhood with others, but by being unable to do anything that requires standing up for themselves. They cannot refuse anything asked from them, simply because they are afraid of other people. Thus their goodness is compulsive, and they then immediately experience resentment of their own behavior. It consists entirely of actions that they force themselves to do (or not to do as the case may be), simply because they are unable to deny or contradict any person, no matter how right and justifiable the contradiction may be.

Compulsive kindness or goodness of this sort is the symptom and the result of inhibited aggression. The person identifies himself with other people so utterly that he feels sure those other people would feel the same anxiety in being contradicted or refused, the same loss of face, the same loneliness and alienation as he himself experiences in these circumstances. The neighbors naturally find such love unacceptable, and the compulsively good person has very few, if any, true friends. He involves himself in situations that make his life a continuous string of resentments. The compulsive goodness harms one member of the society—

namely the compulsively kind person himself to a degree that society regards as criminal when such harm is done to another person. The compulsively good person treats himself as no human being would treat a dog. When he directs himself to do or not do something, he uses the sadistic rigor and harshness that he is unable to use toward others for fear of the consequences of losing control of himself. He often fears himself more than the direct retaliation of others. The remarkable thing about this behavior is that it is generally a question of minor, everyday, trifling matters that are enacted automatically without any forethought. In more serious actions, the person normally prepares himself and makes enormous efforts to overcome his inability and gets a disproportionate pleasure when he lives up to his expectations. Sometimes such a success is carried over for a few days into the rest of his activity and the person is euphoric until the next mistake, which brings with it a deep state of depression. Even the closest of friends cannot account for these changes, as nothing outward has occurred that would warrant such euphoria or depression.

This perhaps too vivid description is designed to illustrate the tendencies of many sensitive and well-behaved people, whose qualities of humility, shyness, and regard for the feelings of others (admirable qualities in themselves, when not compulsively adhered to) exclude the people themselves from those who are to be treated kindly and respectfully. Such people would benefit greatly if they could realize that "Love thy neighbor as thyself" should not always mean that they themselves are *worse* than any neighbor and may be treated accordingly.

The reason for this "lecture" is that in learning new ways of directing oneself, it is essential to bring about optimal conditions for success. There is a way of ordering people about that makes it easy for them to comply. If people realize the necessity for a certain act, however unpleasant, and are invited to it objectively, calmly, they do what is demanded from them with little opposition. If people are bullied into doing even what otherwise is a pleasant thing to do, they get their backs up and refuse to oblige.

Similarly, when directing oneself rudely—blaming oneself for being lazy, weak, clumsy—one finds oneself stubbornly refusing to oblige. Orders to oneself should be given without willfulness, without tension, without bullying oneself, and only for objectively valid reasons. Only children must do things just to obey orders no matter how unreasonable; this is called, by some, learning discipline. But grown-up people must not treat themselves as if they were children. One ought to learn to be as polite with oneself as with anybody else, and to feel just as awkward disturbing oneself with irrelevant problems when doing anything of consequence. One ought to learn that nagging oneself is as bad as nagging one's neighbor—he would not stand for it—nobody, even oneself, responds graciously or willingly to nagging. The more one trains one's willpower for its own sake, and not to do necessary and useful things, the more one becomes compulsive, rigid in mind and manner and stiff in body. The greatest leaders of men, such as Buddha, Confucius, Moses, and Christ, altered the behavior of millions, making them do very difficult things—not by bullying them, but by ordering them in the same human way they ordered themselves. They are admired, even by disbelievers like myself, not for their willpower but for their poised reflective manner. Kind and objective, they had a clear understanding of what was necessary for the men of their time, and they treated themselves likewise.

One has to set about learning to learn as is befitting for the most important business in human life; that is, with serenity but without solemnity, with patient objectivity and without compulsive seriousness. Clenching the fists, tensing the eyebrows, tightening the jaw are expressions of impotent effort. It is possible to succeed in spite of these faults only at the expense of truly healthy joy of living. Learning must be undertaken and is really profitable when the whole frame is held in a state where smiling can turn into laughter without interference, naturally, spontaneously.

The cumulative effect of compulsive teaching has brought about the notion that as long as one can do a thing without sensation of effort, it is not good enough. From early childhood, we are taught to strain ourselves. Parents and teachers seem to receive sadistic satisfaction from compelling children to make an effort. If the child can do what is demanded of him with no apparent forcing of himself they will put him in a more advanced class or add something to his duty just to make sure that the poor thing learns "what life *really* means." That is, trying to do what one need not do in itself, but simply in order to be better than the rest, and one is not supposed to be satisfied unless one really feels the strain of pushing to the limits. This habit becomes so ingrained in us that when we do something and it comes off as it should, just like that, we do generally feel it was just a fluke—it should not be that easy—as if the world were not meant to be easy. And we then even *repeat* the same thing, to make sure this time we strain ourselves in the usual way, so that we feel we really have accomplished something and not "just" done it. This sort of habit is very difficult to eliminate, as the cultural environment is there to sustain it. It is even glorified as a sign of great willpower. But willpower is necessary only where *ability* to do is lacking. Learning, as I see it, is not the training of willpower but the acquisition of the skill to inhibit parasitic action and the ability to direct clear motivations as a result of self-knowledge.

It is perhaps not unconnected with this that all creative people do things in their own way. Painters, mathematicians, composers, and everybody else who has ever done anything worthwhile, always had to learn to paint, think, and compose—but not in the way they were *taught.* They had to learn and work until they knew themselves sufficiently to bring themselves to the state of spontaneity in which their deepest inner self could be brought up and out. Such people are not free of compulsion—much to the contrary. The difference is that what they produce out of the state of compulsion has some value because of the true spontaneous nature of the production.

It is hoped that the following pages will be of assistance to those who want to learn to learn.

ENERGY

Ideas, good or bad, get hold of us if they fit into the general background of the picture we make to ourselves of the world. Modern psychology began to flourish at a time when the thermodynamics theory of heat and the theory of potential were finally put on a firm basis and clearly formulated by some of the most eminent scientists of that time. Thus, the idea that energy can neither be created nor destroyed became more or less common knowledge. Any educated person knew this, and it was quite natural to formulate the libido theory on the same lines, that is, to be analogous with the energy theory. Emotional energy could accumulate, be dammed up; and, as it could not be destroyed, either steam had to be let off or sublimation had to take place. The same background prevails today and some excellent authors, who now see quite clearly the fallacy in the libido analogy, inadvertently make the same mistake with other emotional manifestations—such as aggression.

The energy analogy does not hold good for emotional urges because there is no question of energy here, but of forms of action. Aggression is a form of *behavior,* not an energy. There is no such thing as dammed-up aggression that increases in pressure until the dam breaks down and aggression flows freely. There is no screen to aggression that contains it and allows its accumulation and there is nothing in the nervous system or in any other part of a man where aggression can accumulate.

In the same way, there can be no question of the sublimation of libidinal energy, because there is no accumulation of libido in the form of energy. The sexual glands do not continue to be active, and sperm is not continually formed if there is no sexual outlet. There is a self-regulating mechanism at work here, as in all glandular secretion. There is probably less libidinal tension after a year of abstention than after a fortnight. (There is nothing in long-term sexual abstention that cannot be attended to in a few days or weeks depending on the health and age of the individual.)

When a person has found her emotional security in compulsive humility (that is to say, when her personal experience of the environment was such as to make it easier to suppress all self-assertiveness in order to gain a friendly environment, while standing up for her own wishes became so connected with anxiety that she was unable to do so without feelings of isolation and intense fear), we can, if we choose, see such behavior as if dictated by aggressive wishes. But it is a great mistake to think that it is dammed-up aggression that produces the neurotic behavior. If that were true, then letting off steam, shadow boxing, screaming, shouting, and beating up an imaginary object of aggression (in a room carefully locked to prevent the living subject from accidentally entering) should completely release the dammed-up aggressiveness and produce a new person.

What actually happens in this process is so complex that one can imagine almost anything in it. In fact, an unrestrained expression of aggression does have a relieving effect. This is due, to my mind, not to the reduction of the pressure of accumulated aggressiveness, but to the amount of confidence the person has gained through exercising the function in which she is impotent. All fine cavaliers rode on sticks before they ventured to climb or be hoisted onto a mount. The therapeutic value of any method can be gauged by just this—the contribution it makes to the learning of the function in which the person is impotent.

This contribution might be only a slight increase in confidence, but if this is followed by positive learning—such as the inhibition of some parasitic element in the function, or the clarification of self-direction in performing the action—then further progress may be expected. The importance of discrediting the incorrect analogy with energy now becomes obvious. The accent is shifted onto the item which is the active element and the fallacy of the analogy is exposed. It becomes clear that continuous shadow boxing and release of aggressiveness by chewing carpets will never make a creative and evolving person out of a compulsive, self-effacing individual. (At the same time, it shows that such an initial step may be useful in order to learn the action that will make compulsive self-eradication less necessary for the inner security of the individual.)

The personal experience of each individual does foster the development of certain feelings, faculties, and functions and excludes others. But there is no question here of binding up energy with the fostered functions out of a total available, so that there is no energy left for the others. This can clearly be seen in cases of supposed libidinal sublimation. Suppose a person has excluded a sexual outlet and has at the same time produced creative poetic work in which we can find rich, symbolic, libidinal imagery. At first, the sublimation theory seems verified. But this is only a superficial view. It is enough for that same poet to achieve recognition, to improve her economic position and friendly associations with men—and then sexual activity is almost sure to develop. In a short time she may reach the same level of excellence in her sexual life as in her poetic endeavors, and indulge in both more fully. Taken literally, the energy analogy behind the sublimation theory cannot account for this renaissance without new suppositions of the release of some other source of dammed-up energy.

Functioning in the living organism cannot be likened to energy manifestations in the physical world except in a manner of speaking.

It is much easier to think that each person diverts his attention to those interests that increase emotive security and withdraws it from those that compromise it. The actual choice made by each person depends on the health of her nervous system and its support, as well as on the environment which may reinforce her nervous system in growing and renewing itself, or force it to adopt crippling tendencies and ways of functioning, gradually narrowing and limiting activity to mechanical routine. In the best cases, when internal security has been so undermined that the person loses the incentive to try, for fear of error, failure is unavoidable. Yet in spite of first appearances, we must beware of accepting the facile explanation of dammed-up emotional urges, because it suggests erroneous solutions, through which the learning of the proper use of self is neglected and no real change occurs. We think of insights, of becoming "conscious," and of similar things as sufficient to make a breach in the dam and let the energy flow into proper channels. But these only show us clearly which functions have been excluded from use to the point of remaining in an undeveloped state. And the sooner we get about furthering the apprenticeship the better.

CALLING YOUR ATTENTION

The following words have been given a stricter meaning than is in current usage:

Adaptation of fish to aquatic existence, the adaptation of the bovines to herd life, the adaptation of the polar bear to the color of the snow, i.e., phylogenetic or species adaptation through mutation and selective differential environmental conditions.

Adjustment to the conditions of a concentration camp, adjustment to urban life, adjustment to dance in ballet shoes, adjustment to traditions, to eat with a spoon, i.e., ontogenetic adjustment through personal experience of an individual.

Unconscious urge for affection of the baby, unconscious drive to live of the newborn, that is, drives, urges or other emotional movements that need no personal experience.

Unrecognized is that which has once been cognized and cannot be recognized, which is there and cannot be cognized like the tension habitually maintained in producing speech which has been originally intentionally made or allowed to happen, that which has been learned and has become habitual and autonomic to the point of complete loss of awareness. Repressed is not unconscious yet is unrecognizable.

1. Human Capacity

Intelligence has been defined as the "ability to think abstractly," the "capacity to acquire capacity," the "adaptability to new situations," and the "ability to grasp complex relationships." Furthermore this elusive ability can be defined in many other ways—but we know of none that satisfies everybody. The ability in question is not sufficient in itself even to pass any one of the tests devised to measure it. One may have all the potential "intelligence" to enable one to think abstractly, to acquire skill, to adapt oneself to new situations, to grasp intricate relationships—and yet come to nothing. *A healthy way of use of oneself is necessary to make use of any faculty.* People with mediocre "intelligence" (whatever this may mean), but with a healthy drive for using it, generally manage to achieve what those with so-called superior ability *could* have done, but did not.

Modern psychologists seem to agree that intelligence is an inherited quality; that is, we either have it, or we do not, and we can do nothing about acquiring it. I am convinced on theoretical grounds that the inheritance of intelligence will be discredited. But at present it is of little practical consequence whether intelligence is inherited or not. The truth is, we can improve our ability to think abstractly, to adapt, and to grasp complex situations, simply because most of us have never learned to use any of these abilities to the full.

To illustrate my contention about intelligence not being an inherited quality, let us examine some other human functions, because this is the important point to keep in mind: namely, that intelligence is a way of functioning, and nothing else.

If we tried to find out whether riding horses is an inherited quality or not, it would depend entirely on the kind of society in which the survey would be carried out. In a society that placed a premium on efficient riding, we would find people asserting that Alexander the Great or Attila the Hun were "born riders," that they had inherited the body, the character, that really fine cavalier posture, and so forth, without which no amount of riding could possibly make one into a real horseman. It would be established —by correctly applied statistics, carried out on families of knights and of ordinary people—that there was a correlation between riding ability and the social position of the family. We would find a higher R.Q. (riding quotient) among children of kings, followed in succession by knights, soldiers, town dwellers, and the learned professions.

In our time and society, there is a premium placed on intelligence, and we find higher I.Q.'s among parents of children who have achieved a better social standing. We would achieve exactly parallel correlations, if, instead of I.Q., we compiled statistical data for spending ability on the the same children. In all these surveys the results would prove a clear correlation, which would indeed prove that the correlation methods are correct and indicate a correlation when it exists. However, if we deduced from the high correlation coefficient that the R.Q., or the spending ability, is an inherent quality carried by genes, we would be as near reality as we are when we affirm that the I.Q. is.

Inherited capacities are, on the whole, fairly evenly distributed in the population. We rarely find men with *double* the capacity of the average man—people who are twice as heavy, who can run twice as fast, who have twice the strength of the ordinary man are difficult to come by. The same is true of people having only *half* the average abilities. Intelligence as measured by the intelligence quotient (I.Q.) is no exception. The average I.Q. is 100, but people with an I.Q. of 200 are even rarer than those with an I.Q. of 50.

The enormous disparity in intelligence that we find in men in most walks of life cannot therefore be explained away solely by inheritance. On the other hand, the differentiations in I.Q. that can be experimentally obtained by using various methods of thinking and training lead to a wide range of differences, comparable with and often wider than those attributed to inheritance. I believe that there is no essential difference between what we call a genius and everybody else except that the so-called genius finds the correct method of using himself—sometimes by fortunate circumstances, but more often by searching for it. Once the method is found and the new pattern is clearly presented, many can do as well and often better than the originator of the method.

There is no genius whose followers have not improved on him. Once a better method of using oneself is known—whether in thinking, juggling, swimming, or acting—there are large numbers of people who can equal or even surpass the original discoverer. This shows that the elements necessary for the discovery are latent in each of us; the genius only provides the pattern coordinating these elements into a whole. In other words, the method of using oneself and the urge to do so is what we generally lack. This distinction is very important, because we can do next to nothing about inheritance, but quite a lot to improve the method of use of oneself in order to release the creative urge.

Some of the great intelligences have recognized that their ability was mainly due to their method of using themselves. In his *Confessions,* for instance, Jean-Jacques Rousseau repeatedly insists on his lack of "natural" gifts and attributes all his achievements to his system of using himself, which took him many years to come by. He found his way by trying to read an author without approval or criticism; i.e., without emotional bias. His system was to learn to present the idea the author had in mind as clearly as possible, to the extent of being able to formulate it as well as the author would have liked. After prolonged apprenticeship in this skill, he found that his ability to formulate the ideas of other men clearly and vividly was increasing at a pace with his ability to think for himself. The methods he used before tumbling onto this idea never yielded anything comparable to what he obtained later in life.

Rousseau noted *"Ne rien pouvoir faire à force de trop le désirer"* (while he desired strongly, he could achieve nothing). Many people fail to recognize the true cause of their inability or failure. The cause is very often not lack of ability, but improper use of self—there must not be too little an urge to do, a desire to act, nor too much. Now, we may not be able to influence our inheritance, but we have a large measure of control over our urges and over the means of freeing them from inhibiting agents of which we are rarely aware. We can learn to adjust our body tensions and the state of the nervous system, so that the self-assertive and recuperative functions alternately dominate our frame. In this state of unstable balance, we find ourselves able to enact what we want more expediently.

We may be in a state of inability to enact any projected idea, from writing a letter to loving. Impotent rage and impotent love have a great deal in common. In both, the *desire* to do is excessive, and prevented from expression by extraneous and contradictory motivations of equal intensity. In the case of letter writing, we know we ought to write and yet we do not do so. In all cases of inability to do, there is the feeling of "ought to," which is more pronounced than "want to." The urge to eat, to think, to move, to have sex is due to specific genetic body tensions, but the sensation of "ought to" is a personal habit formed by previous experience. Genetic functions are very sluggish and difficult to alter without drastic and prolonged changes in the biological environment—but that which is formed through personal experience is essentially alterable and, *a priori,* capable of being influenced by a new personal experience.

Sometimes we are unable to enact certain motives because we want them only too vaguely; we feel the sensation of "ought to want" instead of "want." In such cases, we do not enact anything because "ought to" already contains the element of "I do not want to"; the sensations "ought to" or "ought not to" are inhibitory in character.

Our understanding of the functioning of the human nervous system is so rudimentary that any affirmation about its absolute qualities is as valid as an alchemist's affirmation of the use of uranium or even carbon. We consider the nervous system as something that is entirely fixed from the moment of its inception, and only capable of growing in the same sense that a tree can grow, whereas in fact the nervous system is capable of directed growth. The human beings we know now are the result of growth under particular conditions carefully selected to obtain exactly what that conditioning does, in fact, obtain.

The current conception of Man is static, and people who have grown up in an environment formed by this concept are normally incapable of freeing themselves from the limitations woven into their systems. Even the best among us keep on clinging to anything that will justify this static self-concept. First souls, then instincts, then unconscious, then constitution, and lastly intelligence—they must be inherited and therefore fix the ultimate limit of human possibilities. And, of course, the limit is nothing else but the present limitation. I hope to show that the human frame is essentially a dynamic organization, that human behavior is equally dynamic, and that therefore, "human nature" is a dynamic entity made up of some inherited features and of personal experience, and that most of the limitations we encounter are imputable to the personal experiences we are subjected to rather than to inheritance.

2. Spontaneity and Compulsive Action

Words need careful definitions to avoid conveying the exact opposite of what one intends to convey. I am eating because I am hungry; am I spontaneous, or am I acting under the compulsion of hunger? I see or smell an appetizing tidbit, and I reach out for it; am I acting spontaneously, or am I compelled by the promise of gratification? Thus, there is no general agreement as to whether the origin of my urge is internal or external. And, more importantly, no agreement as to whether the action ensuing is spontaneous or compulsive.

In certain acts, we are aware of something resembling "taking off the brakes"; in others, we have to start our executive machine. In still others, we find ourselves acting before we know what we are doing. In general, it is more or less immaterial how we do things—but to the person who does them it is of the greatest importance.

Spontaneity is a subjective and relative notion, and only a trained observer can tell whether a given action is spontaneous or compulsive. It depends on the internal sensation of resistance experienced while acting or inhibiting action. Thus, we may habitually refer to somebody as "Darling," yet experience internal reluctance—which robs the word of sincerity. There will be no apparent delay or hesitation in pronouncing the word; even so, we will consider the action compulsive because of the inner resistance accompanying it. The amount of resistance encountered depends largely on our earlier experience and formed habits of thought. To kill a chicken is to some people as simple an act as to eat it; to others it may be quite impossible to do. If they force themselves to do so, they may find themselves in such an intense emotional state as to be quite unable to eat that particular chicken. Yet for their next meal they may find no difficulty in eating a roast chicken ordered in a restaurant.

These examples though trivial are nevertheless instructive, as they show clearly the importance of personal experience in the formation of spontaneous behavior. Moreover, they show that it is quite usual to have conflicting patterns residing side by side in, so to speak, watertight compartments. However, occasionally circumstances present themselves where the separation between the two compartments must be broken down and the contradiction must be lifted before we can continue to live in peace with ourselves. Spontaneous behavior, as we have defined it, is therefore possible only so long as the environment remains sufficiently unchanged. Under these circumstances, we never become aware of the conflicting patterns coexisting peacefully but never called upon simultaneously.

If we have little experience in solving such conflicts, circumstances may present themselves where we are suddenly faced with a major crisis, while all the people around us who are not personally involved (that is, not conflicted by these circumstances) remain completely unruffled. These internal conflicts, such as love and material consideration, conscientious objection and war, private enterprise and cartels, universality of human knowledge and scientific secrecy, and so forth have no universal solution, for every person's reasoning depends on her personal history and formed habits of thought. What is important to one person is of little consequence to another, and comparisons with other people's behavior are of little help in solving personal problems. More often than not, trying to imitate other people's behavior only complicates the issue and makes finding the right solution for the individual even more difficult.

Spontaneity is indeed a very relative and subjective notion. In species having strong instincts, the individual animal has very little personal say in what it does. It behaves in normal conditions with little internal resistance most of the time, or it is caught up and mauled or destroyed in exceptional ones. In humans, where the bulk of activity consists of learned acts, there appears a kind of activity that is best described as *potent activity*. It is the sort of behavior we encounter in well-matured persons. With the development of voluntary control, we gradually learn to rely on ourselves and decide how much pleasure we are ready to forgo in not complying with the habits of thought and action instilled in us, and how much displeasure we are ready to incur by acting against them. In short, we gradually take the responsibility of our own actions. Short of this maturity, we revert to passive resistance, enacting partly our defiance of the habit and partly our compliance with it. In those planes of life in which our maturity is least developed, we continue acting compulsively; we do (or we do not do) things knowing perfectly well that we want the exact opposite. Under these circumstances, impotence appears. It is important therefore to investigate closely how we learn to act, how internal conflicts arise, and how they are expressed, so that we are better equipped to deal with impotence when it arises.

From the earliest moments of our lives, we can distinguish two sorts of actions: (1) those where we are left to ourselves to work out our own way, as in learning to comply with the demands of our bodies, and (2) those where the adult in charge of us becomes emotionally excited and encourages us to continue our actions, or discourages us to the best of her ability or judgment. There is no clear-cut subdivision of these actions; that is, actions in which we are left to work out our own way suddenly become the focus of adult interference, and *vice versa,* actions that were strictly supervised are just as suddenly left to take their own course. From this process we emerge with (1) a series of personal behavior patterns with which a comparatively low emotional tone is associated and (2) others that are always accompanied with a high emotional tension.

The first actions are performed in their normal setting without any special bias for doing them; we can as easily refrain from them. We can repeat them without any strong feelings one way or the other, or completely refrain from enacting them. They rarely involve hesitation; in short, these are the most spontaneous acts we are capable of, and they constitute the bulk of activity of normal adults.

The other actions—those that evolved under prolonged emotional stress, or those that have been too violently transferred from one group to the other, or those which have never been allowed to stay in one group or the other (because of the irregularity of the adult behavior)—continue to be associated with a high emotional intensity. Children who have always had a lot of fuss made about their food, their clothes, or their looks continue to associate with these things an emotive intensity unless they have learned not to do so. When performing such actions, we become aware of an urge to stop ourselves from doing them. Since the urge *to* enact them is greater than the urge *not to,* we enact them compulsively under an emotional pressure. When refraining from performing them, we become aware of an urge to perform them—they are compulsively inhibited. In compulsive behavior, we are aware of inner tension and resistance; we feel strain when acting the way we do. This strain is always expressed through muscular tension of the muscles of the face, the neck, the abdomen, the fingers, or the toes that can easily be detected if looked for.

Let us examine a crude example. Every child is sometimes lifted briskly overhead. The first time this happens, she blushes, halts her breath, and contracts her flexors—that is, she curls up and prepares to cry. However, most parents do this sort of thing to amuse the child, so they normally give her time to realize that there is no danger in it. The child relaxes, smiles, and if the first trial was not too violent and did not produce an intensely unpleasant sensation, the child will normally ask to be lifted again and again. She finds the repetition more and more enticing for she has learned to contract the abdominal muscles in time to stop the oncoming palpitations of the heart. She halts her breath less and less, and she soon knows how to arrange her body so that she can check the unpleasant sensation. The ability to do so is a pleasant feeling in itself—it is a new experience and the child has learned something.

We can see then how the child learns body patterns that enable her to check and master the onset of unpleasant sensation through experiences in which the child has been allowed to judge for herself the degree of the intensity of unpleasant feeling with which she can cope. She will soon improve on her own performance, and the whole thing will pass into apparent oblivion in the way all experiences of this sort do.

The body has to be adjusted to cope with all excitations, be they pleasant or unpleasant. Some special arrangement of the abdominal cavity and the breath is necessary before we can face being tickled, swung, and turned. If the apprenticeship is not too violent, the response of the body becomes more and more mechanistic, with less and less emotive reaction involved. By and by, we learn to control the reactions of the body until we are able to experience pleasure at being swung or turned, depending on how we arrange our body at the moment.

In the adult state, the expectation of intense sensation continues to provoke us into tensing the abdominal muscles and holding the breath as these help to check the quickening of the pulse and all the other unpleasant reactions of the body in such cases. We fend ourselves thus against the exaggerated intensity of sensation, pleasant or unpleasant. When the expected sensation is unknown, untested, we tense our body sufficiently to be able to cope with it and to prepare for the greatest possible intensity.

In this way we learn to cope with most happenings in our life. The tested, familiar, and often repeated sensations become habitual. In the long run, we stop preparing for them; we do not tense our muscles more than necessary for the accomplishment of the intended action, and we do not hold our breath. But the sensations we have not learned to cope with, and those that we have learned improperly, and (most important of all) the unexpected, untested sensations all continue to produce compulsive body tension. This tension is formed in the expectation of both intense pleasure or intense pain. In either case, the body is in a state of anxiety. This anxiety is present in all compulsive action, and it appears before we can do anything about it. The object of education should be to eliminate these compulsive states and to help the person to acquire the ability for potent action; that is, to be able to control the body excitations and act as in the case of spontaneous action. A clear insight into the general mechanism and the personal history of each individual case, plus the necessary knowledge of self-direction, are a great help in providing satisfactory maturing conditions.

At the root of all anxiety, where education has failed, lies inner compulsion to act or to check action. And compulsion is sensed when motivation for action is conflicting; that is, when the habitual pattern that the person can enact is sensed as compromising the person's security. The feeling of security is linked with the image of self that has been cultivated in the dependence period. Thus, for some people, their good looks—for others, absolute unselfishness, absolute virility, superman ideas, absolute goodness, and all kinds of imaginary, untestable notions, habits of thought and patterns of behavior—have served as a means of obtaining affection, approval, protection, and care. Compulsion is sensed when there is a threat of any of these means becoming ineffective; the person feels endangered and left without any means of protection. When there is objective danger, with no means of defense, the result may be real destruction. In cases of internal compulsion, the only possible result is inner collapse, as there is no objective danger. The anxiety experienced in the face of real danger would normally be experienced by most of us. But the anxiety which is due to inner compulsion has no apparent reason; it is essentially linked with the means of getting security that the person has formed during her personal history.

As the dependence on the adult diminishes, we become more and more potent; that is, we stop acting after earlier established patterns. We feel we can risk applying those parts of our earlier experience that we find expedient and we can reject the others, or try new patterns and are prepared to pay for doing so. In the maturing process we have the opportunity of finding out how far we can go in dropping old habitual patterns acquired during the dependence period. The aim of education should be to help the individual achieve the state of an evolving being; it should make it easier for the individual to sever habitual dependence links, or at least less painful to perpetuate them when judgment demands it. Education that has not achieved this aim is a failure; mature independence then becomes a heavy and tiring task and a continuous struggle against oneself.

People who have emotional difficulties are generally worried whether they are normal or not. They are continuously brought back to this question by the queer and unpleasant sensations that they experience in the instance of enacting compulsively some simple acts that are of little consequence to other people. They tense themselves; their flexor muscles tend to contract and remain contracted for long periods; they feel slightly giddy as if they were going to be sick. They blush or become pale, they perspire for no apparent reason or feel dry in the mouth, they need to evacuate their bowels or bladder without any real necessity for doing so. Or they have a sinking feeling in the pit of the stomach, or palpitations of their heart. Some have the feeling that they are going to faint, that they may lose control, or burst, or a mixture of these sensations or similar ones. People who suffer from some kind of impotence, and especially men suffering from sexual impotence and women unable to obtain full orgasm, will easily recognize in themselves one or the other of the enumerated symptoms. Most of the listed feelings can also be reproduced by strong stimulation of the vestibular apparatus of the ear, quick rotary movements of the head, or intense swinging of the body; sudden lowering or lifting also elicit the same sort of feelings. People who are prone to feel the way we have described do in fact dislike sharp and prolonged rotations, swings, and intense acceleration in general. Sometimes their dislike is so great that they avoid such movements even in their daily behavior, in their gait, and in turning or bending. The highly strung person is recognized by the muscular readiness to stiffen in order to prevent any movement that may produce these unpleasant sensations. She must be ready to check and control her body lest it become involved in the sudden, uncontrollable motion that she dreads.

There is nothing essentially abnormal in all this, except for the seriousness with which it is viewed, and the intensity and constancy of the feelings. As in most disorders, and especially emotional ones, the question is that of degree, and not quality. Intense accelerations, linear or rotary, will always produce intense unpleasant irritation of the vestibular apparatus, nausea, giddiness, and all the rest. The exaggerated sensitivity of some people, and the importance it has in their lives, however, needs further elucidation.

3. Motivation and Action

Urges to essential actions can be traced to body tension. We eat because we are hungry, we rest because we are tired, we dance because we are impelled to muscular activity. In each case the activity produced dissipates and relieves the tension. Most of the essential tensions, like the ones just mentioned, are more or less strictly localized in the body, and we have no difficulty in recognizing them and producing the action that relieves them. There are, however, some tensions which are not so easily identified, and where it is more difficult to produce the action needed to dissipate them.

These other tensions are more diffused. They originate in the higher nervous centers in many different ways and are rather difficult to identify, because the sensation they produce is not connected with a definite part of the body and because they rarely repeat themselves in identical conditions. The sensation of insecurity, for instance, can be produced in relation to so many different parts of the body, in such a variety of ways, different for each individual and different from time to time even for the same individual, that it is not always easy to recognize the tension as related to insecurity. It is therefore very difficult to believe that we are as ignorant as we are of what is happening in us, before the onset of awareness. We generally find some sort of rationalization for the sensation of longing, anxiety, and irritability, so that we need not bother with it too much. When these sensations persist to the point of interfering with the joy of life, it becomes very important to be able to identify the tensions so as to know what to do to find relief, and not just wait for that to happen.

Definite, recognizable tensions motivate our actions. We shall extend the use of the word *motivation* to all actions. We shall therefore distinguish between *conscious* motivation, *unrecognized* motiva-

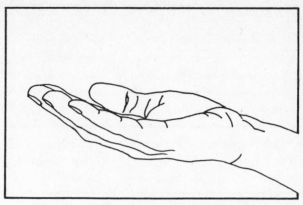

Turn your hand with the palm upward.

tion, and *reflex* motivation, according to the path and origin of the impulses that bring the muscles into action.

Simple actions correspond to simple motivations. In the adult, no act is really very simple. For instance, turn your hand with the palm upward; now turn it with the palm downward. Repeat this sequence half a dozen times with your eyes closed; then open them and turn your hand once more. (Stop reading for a while and try the experiment just described before you know what follows.)

If you were observing yourself, you would have noticed that when your hand is turned with the palm upward your fingers are bent; when your hand is turned with the palm downward, your fingers straighten slightly. So though you were required only to turn your hand, you were in fact enacting something more in addition, namely the bending and straightening of your fingers. This bending of the fingers was not intentionally wanted by you, it was not essential to the performance which you had clearly motivated, and it had no motivated *raison d'être.* Unknown to yourself, you were doing something with yourself. This happens normally in most reflex movements. The weight of the fingers being the same in both cases, the stretch reflex should have acted identically in both positions. Also, the length of the tendons and ligaments cannot wholly account for the difference observed, for in both positions it is still possible to further bend or straighten the fingers.

The main reason for this asymmetrical action of the fingers is that we "habitually" straighten our fingers when the palm is turned downward while taking hold of objects or grasping things. In the other position the hand is clenched most of the time, and the fingers bent, as when bringing an object toward ourselves to look at, smell, eat, or listen to.

The interest of this little experiment lies in that you were aware of only one motive for action, namely that of turning the hand. But you have enacted yet another unrequired movement, which remains unrecognizable partly because it is reflective and partly because of habit. Just for the sake of checking out how much the explanation of habit is correct, try to grip a cigarette or another small object between the index and the middle finger and then repeat the turning of the hand. Your fingers will now more likely remain extended, independently of how your hand is turned. The gripping of the object is now the recognized motivation, and the bending of the fingers therefore needs a conscious new motivation.

Thus, there is a mode of action differing from reflex activity that remains unrecognized because of habit formed through personal experience, but that at one time required awareness and conscious motivation. In reflex movements, we never become internally aware of the motive for action in our body without watching ourselves for a considerable time and knowing what to watch for.

There is a whole series of borderline cases in between these two kinds of action—(1) the reflex action that is a purely physiological property of the nervous system, having little to do with the personal experience of the individual and (2) the one entirely depending on personal experience, that may have become so habitual as to be automatic; that is, difficult to recognize as being issued from a voluntary center. From the point of view of better coordination of one's action, these borderline cases are perhaps the most important ones, as very little attention has been paid to them.

The conditioned reflex theory is now common knowledge. A

healthy animal begins to respond to a quite arbitrary and normally unessential signal—such as a particular noise, the sight of a given shape, a scratch, to a simple lapse of a short time interval—in the same way as it responds to food intake. The unessential signal (conditioned stimulus) must be repeated a few dozen times immediately before giving food to the animal. The food is considered an "unconditioned stimulus," as it needs no previous experience of the animal to provoke salivation and all the other internal processes required for absorbing, digesting, and assimilating food.

It has been proven that the succession of stimuli is of capital importance; namely, the unessential signal must be made before, and not after, the presentation of food if the animal is to be taught to respond to it by salivation as to the presentation of food. It has also been found that an animal in which the higher nervous centers are not in good working condition cannot be made to behave in this way no matter how much trouble one may take to condition a new reflex in it. Thus, in a decerebrated animal or bird, not only is it impossible to establish a conditioned reflex, but all those that may have been established before the removal of the forebrain cease to operate. To abolish all conditioned reflexes, the higher nervous centers must be prevented from normal operation by decerebration; that is, by cutting out the two hemispheres of the brain or by doping the animal with alcohol or with other drugs.

The fact that the higher nervous centers must be in working order before any of the phenomena of conditioning take place is of the greatest importance in understanding the mechanisms of learned behavior, because there is a third mode of action that cannot be accounted for either by reflex theory or by habit formation, although it is usually glossed over or forced into one or the other of the known groups. This third kind of action is particularly interesting because it very much resembles the neurotic response, namely stereotyped action. At first sight such action looks purposeful, motivated, and coordinated. On closer examination, however, the suspected purpose appears doubtful and secondary, because it is either not achieved or achieved with complete indifference. We are then inclined to think that what we initially took for a motivated purpose is merely an arbitrary conditioned signal that is reflectively associated with an unconditioned reflex of defense, feeding, or sex.

A few experiments out of Professor N. A. Popov's work will make the position clear.

Experiment 1.

Thalamic pigeons (that is, pigeons in which the forebrain up to the thalamus has been removed) sometime move in a circle making the specific noise of the normal male courting a female. This reaction can be elicited in the thalamic pigeon by any stimulation such as whistling, clapping the hands, blowing at it, or jerking the cage. But the presence of a female has no effect whatsoever. This stereotyped reaction can be reproduced hundreds of times in a few hours without weakening, and (as stated) by all sorts of stimulation.

Experiment 2.

Thalamic chickens peck the ground around them as if feeding. But close observation shows that they do not pick up the grains, but simply peck and disperse them. If some colored bits of stone are put with the grain, they peck at them as well as at the grain. When a thalamic chicken is resting, the pecking reaction can be elicited by speaking to it, touching it, moving the cage, whistling, or blowing at it. The reaction lasts ten or fifteen seconds and can be repeated without weakening at short intervals, but disappears after forceful feeding of the bird.

Experiment 3.

Two puppies had their cortexes removed at an early stage. They continued finding their food and eating it when it was placed in their cage. They were usually asleep when the food was introduced. The reaction was as follows: movement of the nostrils, licking of lips with the tongue, lifting the head, sniffing around, getting up and moving about until stumbling against the food, and then eating it. This looked like very normal behavior until it was discovered that the puppies would repeat all these same movements in the same order, except the eating, when woken up from sleep by any stimulus whatsoever such as rubbing their noses with ammonia, clapping the hands, or jerking the cage. If the stimulation was repeated after the puppy went to rest, the entire stereo-typed reaction followed over and over again, provided some interval was allowed between successive repetitions.

The full significance of these observations becomes apparent when it is realized that the stereotyped reactions in question cannot be considered as conditioned reflexes for two reasons. Firstly, in intact animals food must follow the conditioned stimulus—otherwise the established reflex becomes weaker and weaker very rapidly and is soon finely extinguished. Secondly, the formation of individual temporary connections in the cortical areas and the underlying ganglia is the basis of Pavlov's theory of conditioned reflexes. In the animals in question, the cortex was extirpated and the reaction continued stereotyped without any sign of weakening, although the unconditioned stimulus never followed. The cyclic character of the stereotyped reactions seems, therefore, to be a property of the lower nervous centers; that is, a complex sequence of acts that can be reproduced as a physiological act. The cyclic character suggests a purposeful action of the kind that we normally associate with a conscious act or with a reflex action to which we ascribe an evolutionary purpose of feeding, protecting, or procreating. Whereas, in fact, the cyclic stereotyped sequence is seen to be a property of the lower centers, which is enhanced by removal of the higher centers of the forebrain.

The newborn responds to many different stimuli by sucking; this reaction disappears immediately after feeding. The conditioning of feeding reflexes is formed out of the inborn property of the lower nervous centers of cyclic stereotyped action.

We often imagine a definite purpose in compulsory stereotyped behavior, because we cannot explain by anything else a sequence of actions that looks so purposefully coordinated. We, therefore, speak of *unconscious* motivation. But the cyclic orderly character may be nothing more than an indication of functional disorder of the higher nervous centers or their fatigue.

The following experiment is instructive in this context. A pigeon was suspended in a special holder, with its legs free. A number of different stimuli, blowing, jerking, and bright light, were tried without eliciting any defensive reaction of the leg to which a recording needle and an electrode were attached. Then for ten days a strong induction current was passed through that leg. After that the previously tried stimuli—which had never been used in conjunction with the current, so that there was no question of a conditioned defense reflex—resulted in strong defensive movement of the leg. Moreover, a conditioned reflex becomes extinguished if the conditioned stimulus is applied repeatedly without the unconditioned stimulus following, while this pigeon manifested the defensive reaction every few minutes for three hours on end without any sign of weakening. Six months of continuous daily excitation did not weaken the response. No weakening was observed after doping the bird with alcohol, which normally abolishes conditioned reflexes.

Thus, we may consider three main kinds of action: (1) the *reflective action* that is innate in our nervous system because of evolutionary experience, (2) the *habitual and conditioned action* that is formed through our personal experience and which needs the inhibiting and regulating influence of the higher nervous centers, and (3) *cyclic stereotyped action* that appears with the weakening of the higher conscious centers. In the reflex action, we never discover any motivation subjectively; thus we cannot feel the contraction of our pupils in daylight. In the habitual and conditioned action, we feel or can become aware of the motive of our action. The cyclic stereotyped action is a mechanical phenomenon of the lower centers, and we should not look for the motivation dictating it, but for the mechanism by which it is produced.

The ideal conscious action corresponds to a clearly recognized unique motivation. The conscious act is *mono*motivated, and the skill of acting consists in acquiring the ability of inhibiting and excluding all the parasitic elements that tend *to enact themselves* by habit, conditioning, and stereotyped motion. Most of the time we fail to achieve what we want by enacting more than we are aware of, rather than by missing what is essential. This is particularly true in learning new skills. One tenses and enacts a considerable number of unnecessary and contradicting elements of action; only later on does one appreciate how much more one did than what was actually wanted. One could swim straight away if one could eliminate all the parasitic acts and perform only those movements that propel one in the direction wished. The expert swimmer produces only those movements that are wanted, and herein lies his skill. His action corresponds to the clear motivation *and to that only.* In the learning stage, a number of habitual and faintly recognized motivations enact themselves. The essential in learning is to become able to recognize these unwanted faint motivations and to discard them.

The importance of having one clear, recognized motivation, and of being able to inhibit or discard those that tend to enact themselves through habitual mannerisms, can be brought home on examining any of our acts that do not bring the intended result— or, better still, those that just barely succeed or are more or less a failure. We will always find ourselves enacting extraneous motivations that are due to habit and formed attitude.

There is, for instance, the person who "asks" for some information (and one wonders at any possibility of, and admires, the simple, impersonal reply). The questioner enacts unrecognized hostility to authority, he enacts provocation, he squeezes the answer out as if to emphasize that his interlocuter has no choice but to answer the question. His question is also more often than not unanswerable in simple and direct terms. He gets the answer to his worded question and not to the intended one (even though that one may be quite easily guessed at by anybody). His action is a failure or nearly so, because of extraneous parasitic motivations that he enacts by habit and formed attitude. His action always produces very similar results, that (1) sustain him in his hostility to authority and (2) are then dissipated by shifting the responsibility onto somebody else, preferably onto some "they." Such a person acts like the learning swimmer—he enacts much more than is necessary for his purpose. He is a "beginner" in correct action, and his behavior is "infantile," as he has not learned adult management of motivation.

In a similar way, we find people enacting guilt, perfection, goodness, searching for approval, and affection, in acts that can best be done without these habitual motivations. Note that all these motivations are neither good nor bad in themselves; neither do we think that the world can be changed overnight, but "our" world, my world, or your world can be *bettered.* The world needs correct action, which is simpler in fact, though not simpler to achieve.

We have seen that the simplest movement we do is of overwhelming complexity from the point of view of what is going on in our nervous system in order to produce it. Bringing a morsel of food with the aid of a fork to our mouth needs prolonged learning before it is done properly. This simple act is made up of an immense number of elements fused together into one act. If one of the elements is considerably different from what we are used to, even this simple act becomes difficult, even impossible.

For example, suppose you are at a public dinner and find yourself using the wrong kind of fork for the dish served. At that instant the act of feeding may become extremely difficult for you to accomplish. The mature adult person in this situation finds no difficulty either in continuing to use the wrong fork or in correcting his mistake. Other people may find their movements so completely disorganized as to make everyone present aware of their difficulty. To produce the simplest movement properly, we need a unique or a dominant motivation.

In the case of man, even the simple act of taking food cannot be performed without having learned to inhibit a certain number of motivations, and without integrating some others into a resultant dominant motivation. The simplest case is when the motive for the act is recognized as one of the periodic tensions of the body segments, as in the act of breathing, and when no contradictory motivation in the body or in the environment foils it. Because of the dependence factor, there is practically no act that we are aware of performing that has no contradictory motivations. Formation of habits is essentially an apprenticeship of managing multiple motivations to form sufficiently dominant ones in each expediency.

4. Resistance and Cross Motivation

We have distinguished two kinds of acts: (1) acts produced in direct response to external stimuli that need not necessarily interest the higher centers of the brain, and (2) acts that do, and of which we become aware. In between these two extremes lie all those acts and movements that are so habitual that we are no longer aware of doing something to produce them. As muscles do not normally contract without nervous impulses reaching them, these different kinds of action must correspond to some difference in the origin, kind, or path of the engendering impulses. The reflex movements are due to impulses from lower nervous centers; they can usually be inhibited by our intention. This is especially true with the striated muscles, which are the skeletal muscles that produce movements. We have considerably less authority over the smooth muscles; that is, over the sphincters (as in the iris, and the anus).

The impulses motivating reflex acts reach the muscles earlier than do those producing intended acts. The reflex impulses have anatomically shorter nervous distances, and fewer relays, to travel from their origin to the muscles. When an intended act contradicts a reflex action—although both have been started by the same event—the reflex impulses arrive earlier, and we feel our body refusing to obey. The reflexively motivated attitude or movement of the body feels as preexisting to us, and we become aware of *resistance.* Habitual acts become in time more or less independent of our intention, and when they are practically automatic the impulses travel through fewer relays and become comparable in speed with the reflex movements. Impulses contradictory to the intended ones, due to these habitual automatic acts, produce the same sensation of resistance. The feeling is as if the resistance were due to something that existed prior to the intended act. We need apprenticeship before we can learn to become aware of enacting that which is sensed as resistance.

The sensation of resistance in action is due to enacting contradictory motivations. Unless there is a sufficiently dominant motivation, we have difficulty in acting properly because the impulses contracting the muscles add up algebraically. That is, when they are not contradictory they add together to make a larger impulse. But when they are contradictory, the larger impulse produces action corresponding to what motivation is left over after subtracting the smaller opposing impulse.

All acts that we perform well are monomotivated. Those that we can manage to perform with considerable effort are more or less dominantly motivated. Those that we cannot bring off are contradictorily motivated by motivations of equal intensity or are ones in which the inhibitory motivation is the strongest.

Thanks to the history of human society, a considerable number of extraneous motivations are formed around each act. It is incumbent on any highly organized society to form the new generation so that it can continue the process of development. And the human social development is favored by the long dependence period of the younger generation, because initially teaching and learning are possible only under the duress of utter dependence.

The richer and more complex the life of a society, the greater is the skill required from the new generation at the moment of taking over, and therefore the stricter is the drill to which it has to be subjected—unless a new and better method of teaching is available. We see in fact that the adolescence period steadily increases. The age for leaving school is now extended to the age at which our forefathers were already heads of families in their own right. We leave school when we are physiologically reaching complete sexual maturity; that is, we are barely weaned of utter social dependence when we are already physiologically mature. Thus, infantile social and economic dependence are maintained forcibly during the period of sexual formation. The situation is therefore inherently fraught with dangers, as at our maturing age we are maintained (from the point of view of independence) in quite unfitting conditions. Little wonder, then, that the sexual function will be hampered in its development in most people.

As could be expected from this analysis, the sexual function is frequently hampered by considerations of economic security (in most cases) and of emotional security (in the worst cases). In general, the patterns of behavior formed during the dependence period prove their worth and adequacy at this junction. If they were rational, the new adult should experience little difficulty in the sexual function—physiologically, psychologically, emotionally, and socially. But if they were not rational, all the errors of education—such as excessive violence and laxity, excessive meekness and aggressiveness, or excessive absoluteness and dogmatism —will show up in this sexual function (the last to mature and in fundamentally adverse conditions).

For example, most young men have been so thoroughly drilled in their dependence period that they will deny themselves, without rebellion, the right to get married because of lack of situation or income. They believe that only a man who earns enough, who can buy things for his wife, has the right to desire one openly (to mention only one of the extraneous motivations that become linked with the main sexual one). When we consider only this one factor, we can begin to fathom the depths and the heights of the obstacles that are heaped up on the road to sexual maturity.

Our civilization makes such drastic and difficult demands of social adjustment that we should not consider frigidity in women and impotence in men as physiological deficiencies, but as the result of successfully achieving a mistaken education. In normal action, the activity that is called for by a body tension relieves the tension. The actions are very specific: to relieve hunger, we must eat; to relieve tiredness, we must sleep or rest; to relieve itching, we must scratch. In the same way, only the sexual act culminating in a complete orgasm relieves the sexual tension. But in all cases of inability to do—such as frigidity and impotence —there are introduced parasitic motivations, the intensity of which is equal to or greater than the motivation of the sexual tension. The person is unable to integrate them all into a suffi-ciently dominant motivation one way or the other.

Moreover, the continual repetition of inhibitory motivations of social origin that operates each time sexual tension arises brings the person to such a state of emotional confusion that she loses the ability to discriminate among the different motivations. That this is possible seems amazing—yet look how many people proceed with the sexual act to prove to themselves that they are adult or independent, or to extort admiration! How many mistake the longing for affection or the need for social power for sexual ten-sion, and proceed with the sexual act to satisfy these cravings! *The sexual act can relieve only sexual tension; all extraneous motivations remain unadulterated.* Itching cannot be relieved by eating a bun, no more than hunger can be satisfied by scratching oneself (though the itching may be alleviated and the scratching postponed if the bun is buttered and jammed). In the same way, it is impossible to satisfy a craving for affection, security, approbation, power, inde-pendence and the like by the sexual act. And those people who do proceed with sexual action when there is no sexual tension, except the tension of habitual extraneous motivations that were mixed up with sex in the course of their individual experience, rarely relieve that tension. They just mitigate it and they find themselves chang-ing one partner after another in the hope of finding one who will do the trick for them. Such people find themselves impotent or frigid, as they try to relieve one tension by the means specific to another. They often vaguely realize that they are not really want-ing sex and decide that they simply are not passionate people, or that they are sexually weak. And so they often drug themselves with aphrodisiacs or vitamins, or some other means alleged to stimulate glandular efficiency.

People find it easier to believe that their makeup includes some physiological or even anatomical insufficiency than to realize the actual situation. Purely anatomical insufficiency is comparatively rare and does not interest us here. The readiness of people to explain their incapacity to do by pointing to their hereditary makeup lies in that, being immature, they shirk responsibility and cling to anything at all that will free them from the task of shouldering it. They also continue to experience guilt and shame and to think themselves wicked and sinful.

These sensations require an internal admission of one's fault before one can sense them. One has to "deserve" the punishment and approve its administration. All these conditions are found together in those in whom the dependence relationship has never been allowed to reach adult maturity. In such people, the power of confession to relieve anxiety resides to a great extent in the fact that the humiliating nature of the procedure is perceived as an installment of self-punishment. Also, the need for approval is partially satisfied by the presence of the confessor. And, finally, the expected, imaginary doom and condemnation fail to happen after all.

Close observation shows that general management of motivation is very poor, and cross motivation is very common. The factors operating to cross motivation in the sexual plane are also at work in all other planes of doing. Feeding, for instance, is so often mismanaged from the point of view of motivation that we find cross motivation in most people. Most boys eat to become or to be "a good big boy." To be good, to be appreciated or loved, to be strong, or to be a he-man becomes the motive for eating. Many people eat themselves to death trying to relieve the tension due to the longing for approval or recognition, or the anxiety due to insecurity. They do not eat to relieve the tension of hunger, but thanks to their faulty habits they mistake one tension for another. Eating as a means of relieving anxiety, insecurity, or longing for approval can hardly be expected to be effective. They go on eating then until the stomach is fully overburdened and digestion so laborious as to become somnolent. The sensitivity of the body is reduced, thinking becomes slowed, all the senses dulled—and thus a partial relief of tension *is* indirectly obtained. The habit is sustained with all the consequences of habitual overeating (on which there is no need to dwell).

The same mechanism is at work in people who starve themselves. Eating becomes a bargaining commodity for obtaining from parents attention, affection, security, fuss; later, it may be used to obtain from others—or from oneself—compliments on one's will-power, slimness, good looks, reasonableness. There is always the motivation of self-denial in order to compel other people or oneself to a desired attitude, as well as a good measure of self-punishment in the ascetic.

In all cross-motivated action there is compulsion, the inner compulsion discussed earlier. The action is *not* specific to the tension, and never relieves it fully. Some tension always remains, compelling a new spurt of action. Hence the single-mindedness with which some people apply themselves to tasks that seem of little consequence to others. Some that we in our ignorance call "very great men" have been made by this process. They acted under compulsion and were miserable all their lives. Many think that this process is essential for great achievements, and that if we eliminated misery there would be no great achievements. *I am convinced that achievement is the result of what is done well and that there is no need for misery to be able to do so. Casting away the contradicting motivations brings out the full vigor of one's ability to do.*

The apparent ability of all of us is far below our latent ability, as contradictory motivation diminishes and tempers most of our actions. There is only a quantitative difference between the potent and impotent doer, but no essential difference in kind. In some cases it is possible to see the latent ability, when the contradictory motivations are eliminated or are contradicted in turn. Thus, under hypnosis, quite ordinary people are capable of feats of strength comparable with and often superior to those of well-trained athletes. In such cases, only the suggested motivation is allowed to be enacted, and so we see the latent potential power unimpeded. But in the normal waking state, only a fraction of the power is available; the internal losses due to contramotivation rob us of the greatest part of it.

My considered opinion is that in general we only use a fraction of our latent capacity in most walks of life. The rest is buried in habitual contradictory motivation, to which we have become so accustomed as to be unable to feel what is happening. Great men rarely have greater capacity than you and I have. They are simply more competent managers of motivation—casting aside all those that oppose or hinder the positive motivation—which therefore stands out clearly. The resultant action is unhesitating, without resistance. With such management Voltaire wrote *Candide* in eleven days—approximately the time one needs to copy out this book in longhand writing.

5. Behavior and Environment

Life, like all processes, must be sustained or cease to continue. For instance, organically, a living body perishes as soon as the process of oxidation ceases. The living organism has evolved and adapted itself to an environment with which it makes a functional whole. Thus, at the present moment there is a close relationship between the total mass of organisms sustained by breathing and the total mass of vegetation having chlorophyll. It has been estimated that the total amount of oxygen in the atmosphere passes through the total vegetative and the total living masses several times a year.

Behavior is to the social environment as organic adaptation is to the physical-chemical world. From our earliest moment of existence, we are molded and adjusted within a given social structure. All human greatness, servitude, and misery are the outcome of this adjustment. From the point of view of behavior, the social environment is the first and last important factor. Even the established organic basis of a given disorder is of little importance compared to the social value of the disorder. Deafness or complete asexuality, such as achieved by castration in early infancy, derive their abnormality only from the fact that the subject in question must adjust himself to a society of beings who need to do nothing in order to hear or to have their sexual identity. In a society, social existence is as important as physical existence. The habits we acquire from earliest childhood, knowingly or unwittingly, prepare us for the kind of society in which the adults of the moment live. The things we do, pleasant or unpleasant, and the things we utterly exclude from our range of action are required of us in order to adjust to the kind of existence they lead.

In an established society such as ours, these inculcated attitudes and responses gain ascendance over our relatively weak human instincts, and it is not unusual for us to sacrifice our organic identity to preserve the social image we have formed of ourselves.

Suppose that a man grew up in an environment remaining permanently unchanged, so that no stimuli much different from those reaching the nervous system during pregnancy ever reached and impressed him. It seems reasonable to expect that the nervous cells would grow and establish some connections, but the functioning of such a nervous system could not possibly have much to do with the environment as we know it. If we try to imagine what the internal life of such a man would be—what the visual sensations, representations, and images *could* be without any reference to the external world—we are led to conclude that he would sense the irritation of the nervous cells but would form no image, no color, no perspective, no contrast, and no brightness. If we imagine the same sort of situation with all the other senses, we conclude that such a person would have the sensations, thoughts, and drives common to us all but in the form of an internal perception of nervous functioning; that is, a purely affectional affair. There would be thoughts without any content relating to the objects, sounds, images, smells, or tactile sensations that are found in the external world around us.

What could a person like that perceive as beauty, beside the reduction of muscular tension? What could his idea of love be, without any reference to those sensations that we cumulate through our personal experience of the external world? We can see that without personal experience, there can be nothing more than an ebb and flow of internal excitation, something of the sort we experience in rage, pleasure, or other affect, emptied of the definiteness derived from our senses.

What could right and wrong mean to a person who has never experienced reward, punishment, appraisal, neglect, affection, or rejection? What would be normal behavior in such a being? Could he be hysterical, poised, intelligent, or dull? What does a person without personal experience mean?

Our imagination itself is so harnessed to our personal experience that we can conceive of nothing outside of it. All we can do is rearrange our experience by playing with the order of events in time and their configuration in space, or similar minor artifices to which we are prone to ascribe originality. Even this conjecture of a person growing up without personal experience of the external world is impossible. We cannot really imagine a person growing without food, without breathing, and the other necessary personal experiences of the world that perforce will produce the kind of being we know through our own personal experience, and who therefore behaves like some man we might have known.

It seems incredible to me that we should have believed for so long in the myth of instincts, in the idea of an innate sense of justice, acquisitiveness, generosity, and the rest of what so many still believe to be "human nature." The first inklings of things belonging to us are probably due to the fact that we clothe our babies and that their clothes do not fit the adult. The baby is thus conditioned without exception, to understand that there are things belonging to him only. In larger families, this universal conditioning is tempered by the arrival of the following baby, and there is a marked difference in the attitude of give and take between people who have grown up in a large family and those who have had no brothers or sisters.

The inherited "human nature" is actually a nervous system with a very wide range of potentialities. The man we know is a nervous system adjusted through personal experience to a given environment, with unwanted potentialities being inhibited by the long dependence period. Thus, all human beings are *potentially* excitable sexually by a multitude of agents such as the sight of breasts, the smell of rancid butter, or veiled faces. In some personal experiences, one of these agents will be enhanced and others inhibited, while in the next experience other selections will be made.

The formation of attitudes, habits, and responses has something in common with ordinary mechanisms in general; *the very principle of functioning limits use to certain conditions only, and excludes the possibility of functioning in others.* For example, the volatility of common lighter fuel is an essential principle that makes ignition by a spark possible. This very quality of volatility causes drying up of the lighter fluid, which makes functioning impossible. Moreover, it restrains proper functioning to a limited range of temperatures—not too high and not too low. The principle of the mechanism also contains and determines its end. Something of the sort can be found in the mechanism of human behavior adjustment.

In some existences, for instance, misery is an essential and vital element, without which life is practically impossible or at least unthinkable. Eliminate the apparent source of misery, and the person will resort to the most ingenious inventiveness in order to reestablish conditions in which the old misery can be enjoyed to the full. Simple change of environment is of little avail—as in the case of the woman who married three times and found to her bewilderment that all three men were practically impotent. The poor woman had a nervous breakdown, bitterly complaining of her bad luck and wondering why she deserved such ill fate. In fact, her attitude toward men and the kind of relationship she looked for with them was incompatible with normal mature virility. The sort of absolute goodness and complete lack of distance between the man and herself, as well as the utter security she wanted to find in a relationship and what she was prepared to do in return for all this, made her into a highly sensitive instrument for detecting and attracting men in whom mature sexuality had been inhibited from the start. Moreover, her behavior would only aggravate their complaint if it were not serious enough already.

A pattern of behavior is a concrete reality. It is gradually formed by the special conditions in which a person has grown up. And each person explores his world to find those conditions into which that pattern fits, just like the duck that heads for water. One cannot live in conditions for which one has not elaborated the necessary means of reaction and over which one therefore lacks the necessary means of influence. *The actual existence as it is lived is a sustained whole in which the manner of action fits the environment in an objective material way, no matter how much suffering it may bring to the person who lives it.* To alter the course of an existence, the whole attitude and manner of action must be changed. An alteration of particular details in the environment or in oneself produces generally only a temporary and irrelevant difference, which moreover fades away in due course, the old process then reinstating itself more or less entirely.

Behavior—like potentialities, inventions, and theories—must be sustained by the environment. Babies cry because there is a response to crying. If a condition arose wherein crying led to the destruction of babies, only noncrying babies would survive in the long run, if that were possible, and there would be no relationship between crying and the forthcoming of attention that is the rule now.

In short, a symptom in behavior is the consequence of obtaining results by the means available to the person, or at least by those he can command best. When security, attention, approval, recognition, or other tension-producing drives become so entangled through personal experience that they cannot be satisfied other than through self-humiliation, self-mutilation, or other perverted means, these means will continue to be employed, not withstanding their destructive effect. The person is utterly unaware of the possibility of obtaining the same ends with any other means and enacts his own with complete conscious approval. When the unwanted symptoms can be shown to be the direct consequence of the habitual behavior pattern, or when the person himself discovers this, the revelation comes as a total surprise.

If we look around us and examine the behavior of children and grown-ups with this gauge in mind, we are not surprised to see that the most queerly ingenious means used almost invariably satisfy their authors. They get what they feel they need even if they do inflict untold suffering on themselves. This is the only way in which they have learned to get what they cannot get by means available to other people.

There is, for instance, that person with a funny voice. It is a fact that whenever he opens his mouth, in the street, on the bus or anywhere else, he attracts attention. (It being understood that his oral cavity and his congenital vocal apparatus cannot account for the symptoms.) I know you will find it difficult, even ridiculous, to believe that he thus obtains exactly what he wants. He himself is unaware of that, I am sure. In fact, you may know that he tries very hard to change his voice; he has even taken lessons of elocution. The important fact is that he cannot change his voice in spite of his efforts and that his voice attracts attention. His symptom is sustained by the environment. Suppose we could make the following experiment: wipe out all human beings around that man. He would need no voice, it could not be compared with any other voice, it could not be funny anymore, it would attract no attention. He would then stop making funny noises. His symptom would die a natural death, and he would have nothing to complain about in this respect.

In practice, however, this experiment is an exercise in futility; it has nothing to do with reality, cannot be realized, and cannot have any bearing on the person's behavior. The important thing is what *can* be done; that is, reality and the facts. And these facts are what we began with, namely, that this person has a funny voice that makes everybody aware of his utterings. To explain the other fact—that he tries to change his voice and cannot do so—we are led to think that the person must make a peculiar use of his muscles without being aware of what he is doing.

We have seen that by changing the environment sufficiently, so that the symptom cannot be sustained by it, the symptom will disappear. We also said that a second method to achieve the same result would be to change the person's response to the environment. When a person has been trying to do this but has failed, my contention is that the failure is due to the fact that the stimulus that sustains the symptom remains unknown. Groping in the dark, his advisors, unfortunately for him, did not stumble onto the real cause, which is usually so *obvious* that we cannot see it even when it is pointed out to us. Because we have to make an effort to understand facts so long as we have our own ideas about interpreting them, our interpretation is equally a mode of behavior, that is, a response that is sustained. If we change our response—that is, if we learn that the explanation we offered is the correct one—we will find no difficulty in accepting it whatsoever.

All symptoms are physical facts; they manifest themselves in a living being and must therefore be evoked by an external or internal stimulus. When the stimulus is new, we are aware of it; when it is an old established habit, we are not. A habit has been *learned,* in the widest sense of this word. To change a habit, we must change the environment so that the symptom is not sustained, or learn a new response to the existing stimuli. To learn a new response, we must know exactly what stimulus evokes the symptom. The undesirable response and its stimulus need not be sought anywhere else but in the physical, factual world, within or without ourselves. Most of the time it is more expedient to change one's own response first before changing the environment, although it may be possible to do something in both at once. As I have pointed out before, behavior and environment are a whole that cannot be subdivided and acted upon separately. The indefiniteness is inherent in the intricate correlation of (1) the individual and (2) the medium of his existence, and only in words can we act on one first and on the other next.

HABIT FORMATION

Our ideas on human behavior suffer from habitual modes of thought evolved in the infancy of human civilization. Either we compare ourselves to other animals without qualification of the differences—which in reality are so great as to make such comparisons completely futile—or we think of ourselves as having souls with innate human propensities that make "human nature" what it is—and that therefore we can do next to nothing to change ourselves.

The facts contradict both of these attitudes. The human being has a very limited set of responses that he inherits. On one hand, we glibly speak of "instincts" when we mean "very early established habits," because we see animals having ready-made sets of responses that are set going with very little individual experience. Calves, kids, and other animals can walk and jump about practically at the moment of birth; human beings take years before they can do so, and some never really learn to do so well. On the other hand we think of "innate goodness" or "wickedness" or the like, when we can watch children growing "good" or "wicked" under particular influences; whereas in fact these behaviors are obviously a learned mode of responding to the environment that becomes habitual.

Living things have only one set of executive organs. Everything we do is manifested through the muscles. In the human being, muscular control is acquired only after laborious and prolonged training. In most other animals, that control reaches adult perfection in a trifling short period after birth, as compared with man. All our acts are, therefore, more influenced by our experience and environment than those of other animals.

We speak of our inherent sense of beauty. We undoubtedly have a potential ability to form such an appreciation, but the functioning sense operates on elements of our personal experience gathered from our personal environment. Gutteral Asian sounds are rarely attractive to the unaccustomed Western ear. But to those who grew up hearing them, they are as pleasant as our "th" or "w," which in turn have little to recommend themselves to an unaccustomed ear.

The muddled thinking we indulge in, borrowing one part of an argument from animal behavior and the other from a fictitious, human, godlike soul, is responsible for more misery than one can imagine.

Mr. X, a man with an excellent technical education, complains of impotence. He finds himself lacking because he does not get an erection at once on seeing his partner. Feeling no erection, he gets anxious and contracted and has to give it up altogether. "Surely," he says, "a normal animal becomes potent instantaneously on the approach of the female."

"On what grounds do you think so?"

"I grew up on a farm, and I observed that in most farm animals."

"Your observation is correct, but your interpretation and conclusions quite false. The bull is excited sexually by the smell of the cow in rut, and if the wind direction is favorable he feels her presence long before she comes near to him. He has no habit of inhibiting his desire toward any female, be it his mother, sister, or somebody else's wife. In man sexual potency depends not only on his physiology but on the habits of thought he has formed. You cannot compare other animals with man and if you do so you set yourself standards that can be reached only in your imagination."

The man was advised to tie a rag with a strong smell to cover the bull's nostrils. This he did, to find that in fact the bull showed no signs of awareness of the female's approach and was now quite "humanly" slow in getting his erection when the rag was removed.

Sexual incompetence results, as do other conflicts, from the imagination's being fed on ideas that have never been tested in reality. The person imagines what is expected of him and thinks that what he imagines is really required. He believes that other people behave according to his imaginary concepts, though he has never had the opportunity to reality-test these fantasies.

The most important factor in removing incompetence, besides learning the proper attitude and the correct directives of oneself, is the intimate realization that human behavior is the result of formed habits of thought, attitude, and control, and that it depends on learning to such a degree that we may consider it to be the *only* important factor.

6. The Power of Dependence and Maturity

Comparisons between humans and other animals are vitiated by the omission of the all-important factor of dependence. We can teach a bear to dance, but we must catch it first and break it in; that is, make it utterly dependent on us for its food and subsistence in general. Without dependence, it is impossible to condition any reflexes in a dog, any more than we can teach a child to speak or have good manners. Education, habit formation, and learning in general are impossible without the initial use of the power of dependence.

A clear distinction must be made between (1) the material or mechanistic dependence of all living beings on the environment that formed the evolutionary adaptation of species (such as gravitation and other physical and chemical conditions of the universe) and (2) the temporary interpersonal dependence that forms the individual adjustment of each being. In the human species, where the child is utterly dependent on parents for a comparatively longer period than are most young animals, the two have become intermingled and therefore a source of confused thinking. Personal adjustment considerably influences the physical makeup of the voluntary control of the body, which therefore differs from one individual to another according to their personal histories. Voluntary control of the musculature is formed mainly after birth, and the conditions to which it is called to adjust itself favor the development of those elements that are used more frequently, and retard the development of those that are left inactive or inhibited.

The complete inability to control voluntary musculature for long periods results in an extremely complex association of the different body tensions into patterns of response that are essentially personal and have (theoretically) nothing to do with the inherited properties of the human nervous makeup. Some of these patterns of behavior are so regularly reproduced that at first sight we are prone to consider them as evolutionary characteristics. Thus, in the adult human, fear of isolation or the anxiety felt at the prospect of being left alone may seem instinctive. But the utter dependence of the human child on long-term adult attention makes it impossible to ascertain with any precision the exact measure of the influence of the personal history of each individual in the formation of these reactions. However, the fact that the parents' state and attitude toward the baby's crying (that is, immediacy of response, and sensitivity) has an influence that can be observed in all children, combined with the frequency with which behavior disorders are traced back to the parental influences of early childhood, makes it quite safe to say that the fear of isolation is a pattern formed under the stress of dependence.

The necessity for adult presence has a decisive influence on forming those patterns of behavior that are called for in relations with other persons. The helplessness experienced by the child when left entirely alone tends to reinstate itself when the pattern is brought into action. The prolonged utter dependence on the adult fosters a whole series of responses and characteristics that are linked with body tensions. The need for attention, affection, approval, reward, and punishment are cultivated thanks to the fundamental situation of dependence. Body tensions make the child act so as to provoke a response from the adult, and the way the adult reacts toward the child fixes the emotional patterns of the child. Out of physical dependence grows the mode of reaction, the attitude or behavior patterns, assuring one's existence and subsistence, one's emotional and social security. The need for security is directly related to dependence. It is not surprising, therefore, to find dependence and the craving for independence in the background of all human activity. In every habit of thought, in every action, it is possible to trace the effects of this factor.

Dependence, being the foundation of all our habits from the

earliest moments of our life, is so interwoven into the texture of our personalities and is so self-evident that it is often difficult to become aware of its potency. In all analyses of behavior disorders, we invariably stumble against the effects of this all-powerful factor.

Theoretically, if we admit that conscious control distinguishes man from a purely machinelike organism, the adult stage should bring with it liberation from all the restrictions imposed by infantile complete dependence. The adult should get free of the fear of isolation in general, let alone the actual infantile experience of fearing being left alone. An adult should be able to act independently of attention, approval, affection, and disapproval. This does not mean, of course, that we should not take into account the effect of our actions on other people. It only means that the old, established responses to certain body tensions should not compel us to react by sheer dint of habit. We should be able to consciously control our actions and let ourselves be childlike if we want to or if it is expedient to do so. As it is, however, most of us never really grow out of our infantile patterns, and we continue to behave in such a way in our social intercourse that the erroneous attribution of our emotional drives to instinctive action is only rarely obvious. In many people the need for attention remains as potent as in their infancy; in others, it is the craving for affection; in yet others, the need for approval or the fear of disapproval become the mainsprings of their entire personalities. Only exceptionally favorable circumstances save such people from painful shocks. They generally find the world hostile and need escapist palliatives that shift the responsibility for their shortcomings onto fate, deity, or other unverifiable powers.

Retarded maturity or arrested emotional development is in itself a result of the dependence factor. For centuries it was in the parents' interest to maintain the fear of isolation and the need for approval and fear over emotional security in their children at the highest level possible, on into their adult behaviors. This tyranny alleviated their own fear of insecurity and assured their subsistence in old age. For generations, and in some countries even today, the well-being of the family materially depends on filial devotion to the parents.

The proper attitude of parents should be the gradual liberation of their children from the servitude that such dependence necessarily brings into being. *The basic emotional patterns—which cannot be avoided, because the dependence of the human child is long and complete—must be intentionally invalidated, instead of being fostered (as they often are even today).*

The child's dependence on the parents gradually diminishes. The growth of the voluntary nerve paths and their connective bundles enables the child to assume responsibility for moving and preserving her own body. Gradually, dependence shifts from the parents to other adults, and finally to society. But the body tensions and the emotional drives that identify them continue to need the infantile means and modes of release unless there is something in the personal history of the individual to invalidate the inexpedient patterns. The dependence influence in all its travesties and forms sustains the habits that make up our very selves, or eliminates those that it does not sustain, in which case they die a natural death. The fullest information about a person contained in one item is the nature of her dependence on society; that is, the way she assures her subsistence. To know whether someone is an artist, a tailor, a stockbroker, a prostitute, or a thief gives more information about her than the most detailed description of her inherited physique, the color of her eyes and all the rest of it. Without this information, a person is as fictitious as a screen character. Escapism in all its forms consists, invariably, in cutting out the idea of one's own dependence from one's mind.

The French paleontologist Cuvier said that if you can recognize one tooth of an animal, you can reconstruct the whole animal. To have canines like those of a tiger, the animal must be predatory. It must be swift, it must be mobile, it must have a meat-digesting alimentary tract, and it must live in regions where there is prey. What is true on an evolutionary scale is even more so with us because our preadult period is often as long as a quarter of our life span. Thus, our feeding habits, our social habits, our sexual habits, our ideas about freedom and whatnot are all what our history of dependence has made them to be. Whether you were left to cry before feeding, or were fed at once, or even before you wanted it, has a greater influence today on your relations with your husband than do your looks, your stature, or the color of your eyes—or his. For the habitual response formed by your mode of adjustment to dependence is the only response you are capable of that feels right to you. Thus you create again and again the circumstances in which that response is sustained.

But all this holds true only in the domains of activity that have not matured. We do not grow all at once and uniformly; some parts lag behind the others. This kind of partial development becomes more and more noticeable with time. The original trends enforced in the personal history of adjustment to dependence often exclude further development in certain domains. The effects of these patterns of behavior make themselves felt very conspicuously with every new experience.

In general, the later the new patterns of doing are called into action, the greater our tendency to use the old, established ones with as little change as possible. Because of this, sex relationships and the social function and adjustment of people are the two domains of activity in which maladjustments are the most frequent. Until very recently, education was so dogmatic, and people were so sure of what was good for others, and the ultimate object of life was so obvious to them that they did not hesitate to use the dependence factor to exclude most personal spontaneous tendencies. Little wonder, therefore, that so many carried on their relationships with mother and father into their attitudes toward the opposite sex. Moreover, there was comparatively little harm that came to light, as suffering was generally accepted (because of original sin) as the deserved lot of the human race. Also both sexes had the same hindered emotional development, so that they found in each other corresponding immature behavior, and misfits were probably rarer than we are inclined to think.

In my discussion so far, the human being appears rather like a glorified .nachine, having little say in what is being formed in it. Yet, we cannot fail to observe activity that seems to emanate from the person herself, even in complete contradiction to patterns that were formed under the stress of dependence. This spontaneous activity is observable most of the time in domains that escaped the rigor of dependence and were allowed to reach mature functioning.

Maturity is not a state that is reached and then maintained by itself. It is a way of doing in which patterns of behavior formed in the period of dependence are no longer enacted as the only possible way. During the dependence period, a large number of patterns and modes of action are excluded from normal usage. Some of these banned modes may also be rejected by the mature person, but the reason for the rejection is now deliberate—even though to the immature person rejection by habit also seems quite deliberate. A means of detecting whether the rejection is deliberate, or only appears to be so because of the strangeness of the alternative, is to try to admit the new pattern and follow oneself enacting it. The mature person does not shrink away from the idea and feels no aversion or special excitement at *the thought* of enacting what she thinks she should not and will not. There is no sensation of compromised security.

To conform with the adults' requirements or not, in the dependence state, involves the risk of compromising security. The attention and affection of the parents, their approval and care, are the only means of subsistence, and the child will do everything for that. Conforming with what dependence happens to impose, the child learns to associate security with approved activity. Without maturity—that is, without the ability to break up earlier experience and use only those elements of it that are expedient for the present moment—the dreadful sensation of insecurity arises even at the admission of the possibility of an action that would have compromised that individual's security in childhood. Anxiety is sensed, the flexor muscles contract, especially those clenching the fingers and the lower jaw, the extensors lose their tone, and the head lowers.

We shall see later in greater detail how our habitual activity is formed as a means of avoiding precisely this dreadful feeling of anxiety. As it is, there is no shunning the difficulty. Anxiety must be faced at one moment or the other, and responsibility shouldered if we are to become mature, evolving persons. Without these two preconditions, it is impossible to reach the state of spontaneous action in which we feel complete self-realization. And life without this is hardly worth having. The dependence relationship in which we are given a sweet if we are good girls and boys, in which we have to acquire the right to live by complying with somebody else's desires, must be completely eliminated before a society of creative and evolving beings will be formed.

7. Reward and Punishment

The concrete form in which the child's utter dependence expresses itself is the change in the surrounding emotional atmosphere that every move and every change in his body produces. The attitude of the adult is continuously either approving or disapproving. In the first instance, the child hears soothing noises, feels caressing handling and his body being moved in round, soft curves. In the other instance, the child hears harsher noises, feels rougher handling and his body being moved in a more jerky way, with sharper accelerations and changes of direction. A baby is extremely sensitive to sharp movements. A few minutes after birth, at a sharp lowering of his body the baby's flexors will contract and produce a whole series of changes that express anxiety (this continues to be true for the adult). The child thus soon learns to associate pleasant sensations with some of his acts, and disagreeable sensations with others.

The mere presence of the adult, the all-powerful adult, gives the child a sense of security; his withdrawal evokes the feeling of abandonment; being left alone means utter helplessness. The friendly attitude of the adult gives the child his sense of affection, and withdrawal of the friendly attitude evokes the sensation of loneliness. These sensations are expressed through bodily tensions and are the most lasting experiences, although we are normally unaware of them. With frequent repetition and intensity of affect, they become in the long run so linked with attitudes and internal states that it is difficult to ascertain subjectively which comes first —the internal state, the attitude, or the sensation.

If the adult shows constant regard, the child forms the habit of looking for approval for each action. Without approval forthcoming, the child feels abandoned and lonely and retires into himself. You probably know people around you who need attention, compliments, and encouragement after the slightest effort. Without these expressions, they become depressed and apathetic.

To a certain degree, these habitual reactions remain potent in every one of us. Even "great men" suffer from not getting the approval they expect. The drive for honors, medals, and titles is the normal manifestation of the habit of getting approval in child-hood. The horse that has won the Derby cares much less for the approval of the spectators than that of the jockey—without whom the horse would have been able to run a little faster. But horses too can be conditioned to expect a piece of sugar after their per-formance.

Every one of the sensations mentioned is very weak to begin with, and only long practice gives them the potency and constancy that we find in some adults. By and by these sensations become linked with our habits of taking food, then with other actions such as body carriage, gait, and finally our sexual attitudes and our attitudes toward work.

In every state of depression, mild or serious, we can distinguish one or a mixture of the many forms through which our prolonged dependence on the adult expresses itself. In one it is approval, in another security, in a third affection, and so forth that is needed to relieve the tension that produces anguish.

The great advance in understanding mental states made in re-cent years is mainly due to psychoanalysis. In psychoanalytical practice, the person is led by a special technique to work through unconscious material back into his own history and to find emo-tional relief from the old incidents in the present, when his depen-dence on the adults of the past is either nil or greatly reduced. He can therefore face the old incidents without the stress of depen-dence, and he has a chance and a choice that he never knew before. The violence of his emotions can be abated; he can work them through and alleviate them.

Gestalt therapy puts the stress not on bringing up the uncon-scious material, but on making the person aware of the role played in his life both by each of the sensations we have mentioned and by some others. Starting from the present, the person is led back into his own life history and brought to realize how much his actions were motivated by these emotions, to sort them out, and to guard against them in the future.

The initial attitude of the adult, changing from approval to disapproval (which is expressed mostly by the way he controls himself rather than by his intended action on the baby), gradually evolves into easily recognizable moves. Concurrently, the hurts caused by the inanimate world also increase in intensity; the child falls, or burns himself. These are frequent occurrences and are part and parcel of the individual adjustment to the environment. Punishment in itself is of little harmful consequence if the learning process has not been distorted by too intense an emotional atmosphere or too capricious and changing an attitude (in which case the child cannot find any order to which he can adjust himself, but on the contrary finds that his behavior produces conflicting reactions, now producing the expected result and next the exact opposite).

If a child burns himself he cries and learns not to touch fire again. He may need more than one such lesson, but these rarely cause any lasting emotional behavioral disorders, painful though they may be. The same punishment inflicted deliberately by an adult may be sufficient to distort the entire process of adjustment and leave an indelible mark on the mind of the child. While a child may fall and break a leg, he will be jumping and running again before long. But if beaten by his father to the same point of grievous bodily injury, the entire social adjustment of the child may be distorted. The mechanistic punishment of the physical world, such as the burn that follows touching fire, is regular, consistent, and immediate. One can adjust oneself and learn to avoid it. The child soon learns to associate the punishment with his own act; test it, appreciate it, and avoid it, or accept a bearable measure of it. Such punishment does not disturb the balance of mind and has rarely any lasting effects.

However, punishment from the hand of an adult is rarely so immediate and so consistent that the child can readily associate the punishment with his own action and establish a casual link between them. Moreover, simultaneously with the punishment his security is compromised, so that not only does he feel the physical pain but he also feels left alone. The anxiety is so great that he can compel himself to kiss the punishing hand if the parent insists on this. *The loss of security is a greater anguish than the pain of punishment.* The compromise of security distorts the lever with which the adjustment to reality is made, because it makes the dependence relationship frightening, and therefore destroys the ability to learn.

Punishment that undermines security is unhealthy. The dependence relationship becomes overstrained, and the means of education are destroyed. The child is forced to rely on his own means to assure his security, at a stage when those means are practically nil. The result cannot be anything but detrimental to future adjustment.

However, the punishment that is at the bottom of most future trouble is the most innocent in appearance: the *threat* of punishment is more effective than actual punishment, provided it can be maintained; that is, provided that the threat remains active. Herein lies, in effect, both the advantage of such threats and the seed of possible disorders. The adult finds it easier to impress the vivid imagination of the youngster than to organize himself to corrective action. The efficacy of threatened punishment is that the child is unable to test the truth of the threat or to ascertain its real effects. Such threats are as effective with the immature adult as they are with the child. A threat is essentially a means to control through fear, not a positive constructive tool. A threat almost always achieves its aim—but unfortunately it often does much more than that.

In mechanistic real punishment, the child can appreciate the degree of inconvenience and decide to accept the pain or displeasure if the gratification bought with it is worth it. A promised punishment that cannot be tested creates the inner conflict of indecision. The drive for action is not impeded directly, the dreaded punishment is not real, and the child is constantly impelled to test it and find out for himself how far he can really go.

Thus, for example, if a child is told that he will never be a man if he plays with his sex, that he is wicked, that he will lose his memory, that he will go to hell, that he will never be able to have children of his own, that he will die in the gutter and so forth, he cannot be sure whether this is so or not. His disturbed imagination dwells on these threats, and tries to figure out whether the promised punishment is forthcoming or beginning to manifest itself. The prohibited act is, therefore, repeated not only as the natural means of releasing body tension, but also with the anxious expectation of impending disaster. As he masturbates, the child naturally becomes aware of vascular changes taking place in him. Palpitations and cold sweat thus become associated with the feeling of impending doom (that he expects to descend at any moment). The body changes suggest that the punishment is real. He is now sure that his fears are well founded, and he resists the temptation until the original natural body tension, for which he is not responsible, increases sufficiently, and the same thing is repeated all over again. He is thus convinced that he is really wicked and that he deserves what will be coming to him. There is nothing he can do about it, and unless a drastic change in his environment takes place, nightmares and other difficulties soon hamper the vitality of the child to a marked degree. Many immature adults also continue in the same way, not knowing a better answer, and are just as frightened as the child in question, and likewise remain in a perpetual state of conflict.

Fortunately, it is not enough to make one mistake to create such a vicious circle, unless the first incident is of real dramatic intensity. Instead a considerable number of events in which the child's imagination finds sufficient similarity must occur before harm is done. Soon enough the growing mind finds weaknesses in the parents, and doubts about the validity of these and other parental assertions help the child to regain balance.

The efficacy of promised punishment lies in the fact that imagination is called in to make the time interval between the action and the onset of the imaginary punishment short, consistent, and never failing, just as is the physical pain or discomfort that follows faulty action. Therefore, the feeling of guilt develops rapidly to a high pitch of intensity. Once such a pattern is established, it will normally persist even though the specifics, that is the particular details, may change. A pattern or attitude of behavior has been formed that will run like a frayed red thread throughout the fabric of the person's life.

THE ABSOLUTE AND THE EXPEDIENT

We often speak of objective proper behavior; that is, of a non-subjective attitude toward the outside world. In reality, however, there is no such thing as a truly objective attitude. Even the most impersonal decisions are dictated by our emotions; it is only a question of degree. We consider ourselves objective when we are not aware of any exceptional tension at the time, which only indicates that there is no contradiction in our emotions, that the situation is so familiar to us that contradiction has lost its power. But in reality there is nothing that we know with absolute certainty that warrants acceptance without contradiction. The things we do accept with utter confidence are simply those which we have been accepting habitually and for a long time without feeling the contradiction in them. The father who frightens the life out of a child because it has been playing with a part of its body a few inches below the belt is so sure that he does the right thing that he thinks he is being really objective, and then tells his child things that are as remote from reality as can be. *There is no objective truth; and we are only more or less subjective at the best of times.*

Proper behavior has nothing absolute about it; it must fit the situation in the particular environment and time of the person. In other words, it is expedient, and only a matured person—that is, a person capable of dissociating past experience into its component parts and then using those that fit the present circumstances —is capable of such behavior. Absolute objectivity is impossible in practice, as it is the person who is the sole judge of his behavior and the propriety of his judgment depends on his personal experience of the world.

We are taught to tell the truth. But the truth is a subjective judgment. It varies even in the same person with his personal experience. The defintion of truth that we teach to children would bring any aware adult to wish himself dumb for all time. The truth we demand from children makes it expedient, in their state of utter dependence, to lie, and all children do lie in order to preserve their security. They cannot afford to lose parental affection, and will deny the prohibited act they have done. Under these stressful circumstances, it becomes the truth for them. Now, it goes without saying that a sufficient measure of commonly accepted standards is indispensable for the smooth running of any organized society, and that there is no question here of justifying deliberate lying. What we are concerned with is the understanding and possible removal of morbid conditions in persons who have been led to accept in their childhood certain half-truths as divine precepts, and who have never tempered their convictions by testing them in reality. These are people who feel they are wicked; they accuse themselves of being unable to comply with what they have accepted as an absolute right. They believe themselves guilty, they *know* they deserve punishment, and they mete it out to themselves accordingly.

We can be very ruthless in abusing the utter dependence of a child, teaching him absolute purity, absolute honesty, and so on when we very well know that there is only an expedient truth, an expedient righteousness—just enough to make a given social order acceptable to the majority of people.

We have painted a dark picture; unfortunately it is often a true picture. As mature people, we can trace the working of the same mechanism in our own behaviors, which have been tempered by experimental testing of reality. Normal adult behavior admits only such degrees of right or wrong, such measures of moral and immoral, selfishness and wickedness, as are expedient.

8. The Origin of Faulty Posture

Every one of us thinks he or she can tell a good posture from a bad one, just as we feel we can tell a madman from a normal person. Roughly speaking, we are right in thinking so, and we can pick out both the extremely bad ones and the extremely good ones without hesitation. But if we want to distinguish between good postures, or to improve postures, we find widely disparate opinions even among the experts.

First, the idea of posture itself is fairly new, and in most minds *posture* and *position* mean the same thing. *Posture* is misleading; it suggests fixity as much as position. For example, we say someone has a nice posture when we mean that she stands straight; that is, vertically, she stands as high as she can; in other words, she has assumed a straight vertical position. Well, one can assume a good position while having bad posture, because posture is concerned with the way the good or bad position is achieved. *Position* describes the location and configuration of the various segments of the body. *Posture* describes the use of the entire self in achieving and maintaining this or that change of configuration and position. Posture is therefore describing action, and is a dynamic term. One can slouch, lower the head, and adopt the most awkward position in good posture and assume the same position in very bad posture. *Posture* relates to the use made of the entire neuromuscular function, or more generally, the cerebrosomatic whole; that is, the way the affect, the motivation, the direction, and the execution of the act is organized while it is performed. *Posture* must, therefore, be used to describe the way the idea of an act is projected and the way the different segments of the body are correlated to achieve a change or maintain a state. A cripple may have excellent posture, although the positions he assumes are all abnormal.

To have a good posture, therefore, it is necessary to be skilled in the use of the mechanism for projecting action patterns, to have a good configuration of the body segments and a coordinated smooth control of the muscles—not simply to stand in one particular way or to sit nicely. The incongruity of the term *posture* used to describe a mode of action is quite obvious, and it is regrettable that its use is so widespread and so well established.

The clear definition of the term *posture* helps in understanding the whole problem of bad and good posture. The most common bad use occurs when we are in rage, in terror or extreme emotional stress. Violent emotions produce a wide-spreading excitation of the muscular system and make fine control impossible. The aim is then achieved by sheer expenditure of energy, and no precise delicate action is possible. In such states of intense emotional excitement, we are unable to see alternative ways of performance; we act under inner compulsion. Bodily, this expresses itself through a generalized muscular contraction within which the violent action that we may perform is only a small part of the total effort. The purely mechanical efficiency is also very poor.

The common association of good posture with poise—that is, mental or emotional tranquility—is in fact an excellent criterion of good posture. Neither excessive muscular tension nor emotional intensity is compatible with good posture. Good posture means acting fast but without hurry; hurry means generally heightened activity that results not in faster action, but only in increased muscular contraction. Good posture means using all the power one possesses without enacting any parasitic movements.

Faulty posture can always be traced to those factors that cause increased emotional tone. This happens every time we perceive a body tension, and the means to release it are not available. Bad posture is the externally observable physical counterpart of internal conflict or contradiction. It is cultivated during the dependence period when the child is called on to perform acts for which she has not the means; that is, when she is induced to act by heightening her emotional tone and not *spontaneously*, in the sense we have defined that word earlier. If the child is goaded to stand up or walk before she has completed her crawling apprenticeship, she complies for the gain of affection and approval. She stands up or walks with unnecessary tensions, and these acts become associated with a sense of effort and with a configuration of the body segments compatible with insufficient power in the muscles of the pelvic joints. She will need corrective influences to resume normal development, or she must wait for her last chance when the dependence relationship slackens and therefore her integrative conscious control has grown sufficiently to assume direction of herself. But of course, at that point the formed habit may be so entrenched as to exclude any possibility of change in behavior. In such cases the infantile posture will be perpetuated, and maturity impeded.

FAULTY POSTURE AND ACTION

Faulty posture and behavior arise in a normal way in normal children if the end to be achieved is beyond the means of the child. People slouch or tense their bodies unnecessarily not because there is some nervous deficiency in their systems, but because their means were insufficient at the moment of facing the novel situation. Our dependence on others is so great that we have to comply with what is wanted or expected from us, or else we lose parental affection, social approval, and our means of subsistence. At different stages of our existence, each of these losses means isolation from the habitual environment—which is tantamount to self-destruction. As children, we cannot afford to displease our parents to the point of our complete rejection, any more than we can afford to brave the world beyond certain bounds. Our security demands the performance of what is expected of us, and we have to do it whether we are able to or not.

Faulty posture always expresses the emotional stress that has been responsible for its formation. The most frequent and observable one is the stress of insecurity in its different aspects, such as hesitation, fear, doubt, apprehension, servility, unquestioning compliance—and their exact opposites.

If we observe the carriage of people in the street, we find that one person walks as if he had no right to breathe the air without securing someone's permission; and in fact he does hold his breath most of the time. He has to justify his existence by being good; he has to earn his right to breathe. He is unobtrusive, but all tension; his voice, his movements, and his whole demeanor show the conflict between his desire to live and his inner conviction of his inability to live up to and perform what he himself has accepted as the norm of what he should be able to do.

Now, here is a woman passing. At every step you see her cheeks vibrating slightly, and if you observe closely you notice hardly perceptible jerks of her head and the alternate contractions of the muscles at the back of the neck. She walks very "straight"; if she had swallowed a yardstick, she would not walk any straighter. She is as stiff as a poker, and all her demeanor cries, "I am straight." If she were not straight, she would have no right to live. She is just as insecure as the first man; her straightness is just as compulsive as the former's servility. They have both learned to direct themselves so as to comply with what was expected of them; they both have inhibited their spontaneity. There is little need to multiply examples; it is sufficient to stand for a few moments at the window or in the street to see the greatest possible variety of such deformed human frames.

It is quite erroneous to think, as some posture teachers do, that all the people in the world are wrong and do not know how to use themselves. And it is totally incorrect to think that a bad alignment of the body is the cause of the ailments that accompany such configurations. There is no ailment that is due directly to an excessive protrusion of the chin except very local, minor strain in the articulation of the head. But the process that has produced such a permanent contraction of a voluntarily controllable group of muscles is of fundamental importance to the structure of the person in question. Obviously, then, the lifting of the head, even if maintained forever afterward by another voluntary contraction, would make no difference other than in local correction. The important thing is the voluntary contraction that remains permanent.

This wasted effort shows that the person had to produce it in order to comply with what she felt was an absolute necessity. The faulty posture was the best way in which she could produce at the moment what she had directed herself to do. It was the best posture at that time—and it still is, if she has learned little since.

In the course of growing, every one of us has to learn not only the exterior world, but the use of our own body. Thus we all get toothaches, we all vomit, we all get prune skin stuck to our palates, we all get pieces of food that go into the trachea instead of being swallowed, we all wet our beds, masturbate, are constipated, fall, hurt ourselves, have our first nocturnal emission or our first menstruation. These are only a few of the happenings that we find in ourselves, and we have to learn their significance, how they feel, and what to do to ourselves to cope with them or to check them. They are all very frightening when first experienced, sometimes terrifying. And in the end all depends on the parental attitude— on how calmly, friendly, ostracizing, incriminating, or soothing they are—as to whether we will learn to face pain, and difficulties, without losing control or being overwhelmed.

To combat the onset of fright (to control the onset of nausea, of swooning, of losing consciousness, of choking, of palpitation— in a word, *anxiety*), we all work out our own ways of holding our breath, of tensing our abdominal walls, of tilting our heads, or stiffening our pelvic joints. That is to say, we acquire our individual manner of doing our personal posture. The manner of projecting the idea of action, the way of motivating and enacting our motivation, the way of rearranging the different body segments, and the way of leaving them after an act is performed—remain our own. They can be detected in our way of doing nothing, our way of refraining from doing, our way of thinking, walking, sitting, gripping or letting go, speaking, or having sex. The unnecessary tensions are only unnecessary in ideal—that is, nonexisting—man. The bad postures we encounter are what they should be and would be if the life experience were to repeat itself. Only the process of maturing and the liberation of the affect associated with each action and situation will make any actual difference in the manner of doing, not changing any particular detail of the configuration of the body.

Some special difficulties are common to all of us, thanks to the family order of our society; namely, our children belong to their parents, who normally take the credit or the blame for them. Because of our prolonged helplessness, we will always have to depend on some adults, whatever the organization may be in future. So the remedy is in furthering our maturity when our emotional dependence slackens through greater physical and economic independence. Otherwise, we will always have to allow for the fact that every act has not only (1) the normal physiological and mechanical difficulties to be overcome through learning, but also (2) the ever present adult whose approval must be sought and met. All these normal conditions make it practically impossible to learn anything without linking with it an affect, a sort of a third eye, which watches our mobilization of means and reinstates the original corrective influence in most details. The result of all this is that we screw ourselves up to do things and thus come to associate with all action a sensation of effort. The internal resistance then becomes part and parcel of the action, and a necessary component to perform it. How many people can use a pair of scissors, especially if they are not perfectly sharp, without producing all the contortions of the face, the tongue, the shoulders, and abdomen that originally they had learned together with this action? And, in fact, at the time handling scissors was really beyond any child's reasonable ability, in view of the size and the form of scissors being designed for an adult hand.

Faulty action, unnecessary tension, caricature, and holding of the body are not bad in themselves. When we adopted them, they met with our entire wholehearted approval, and with the approval of those who, not knowing any better, appraised our efforts and helped to make us what we are. To destroy these bad habits of use of self without providing better substitutes is not only difficult but foolish.

The picture we have drawn of the working of the human frame

leads one to believe (1) that we are simply passive reactors to what is happening around us and (2) that what the child is going to be, seemingly depends solely on what happened to her by design or circumstances. The inevitable conclusion seems to be that if a certain pattern has recurred too often or too violently, there is nothing we can do about it except sympathize with the unfortunate person.

This is true if we make no use of the opportunity that the growth of our body and its nervous system offers us, but instead continue to perpetuate the old manner of behavior formed under stress of dependence, without availing ourselves of every change in our economic independence to change our attitudes and free our motivation from the handicap that impedes it. This passive approach—which we have followed only in order to analyze and to underscore the importance of environment and of its unity with every being in it—must not obscure and push into the background, as it often does, the active constructive means at our disposal; means that to some degree are at work in each person.

True as it is that the consistency and the intensity with which the environment acts on the individual are factors of paramount importance, it is not the whole truth. Most people have been punished by their parents who, in good faith, used sometimes proper and sometimes unhealthy methods. It is a fact that most of us are a bit queer in one way or another, and each of us has one corner in ourselves that should not be touched lest we lose control and behave neurotically. But it is also a fact that a considerable number of people subjected to roughly the same conditions achieve nevertheless a high degree of mental balance.

In behavior, however, what matters in individual cases is not what most people do, nor the statistical average, but the individual personal experience. And in any case, our analysis has left out one of the most important factors—*the integrative power of the nervous system.* This power enables the individual to control the impact of environmental influences, to discard the ones she has not learned to cope with and does not intend to learn, and to select among the multitude of possible spontaneous or automatic responses the ones to be enacted. This process is maturation. And if it has been interfered with so that it never ripened sufficiently to enable the person to assume entire responsibility for her own direction, then infantile behavior is paramount and compulsiveness is the rule.

The complex structure of human behavior and its dependence on the environment must not be overemphasized; otherwise, the integrative capacity of our nervous system is barely recognizable and very often completely ignored, as if it played no role in the direction of ourselves. We are often presented as mere playgrounds for the body tensions, environment, and circumstances. Indeed, this picture is often correct, since the normal ways of "education" arrest development in most planes of emotional motivation except those few that are sustained by our ways of life, so that we make the mistake of taking the present and past situation as the norm of human possibility. The greatest difficulty encountered in attempting to break this vicious circle and find the road to maturity is the deeply engrained, erroneous notion that a person is what she is born to be, and that it does not matter what she does because she will always remain what she is. If a person astonishes us by her achievements, we at once decide that she always had it in her and neither she nor anybody else had noticed it. The amount of labor and inner struggle, the lifetimes of learning, and all the woman has done are discarded as of no consequence. What a woman does seems to us to be of much less importance than what she is. With such contradictory nonsense, we continue to believe that a person is, for example, "born" honest, strong-willed, decent, a pilot, or an announcer on the radio—and very soon we will discover some "born" atom bomb droppers, who know "by instinct" where to drop them.

As soon as we realize through our body experience that changes of a fundamental nature can be wrought in us—that there is no such thing as a personality without an environment and no behavior without interaction between them—the road to maturity is open. Ignoring the environment and the properties of the frame growing in it, we find ourselves in blind alleys every now and then, and see no way out. We then ease the qualms of our conscience by clinging to ideas that justify our impotence—souls, inheritance, predisposition, the unconscious—in fact, any notion that will leave us to suffer our indolence in peace. Wars are then not due to human action, but to *"human nature,"* which is, "as everybody knows," inherited and therefore cannot be altered without ceasing to be human nature. And we will therefore continue waging wars whatever we may do. The truth is, wars are produced by human beings in the same way as they adopt wretched postures. Both are necessary and serve a very useful purpose so long as we have no other means of achieving the necessary ends.

Just like the person who adopts a crippling use of her body when confronted with a task for which her previous experience has not equipped her, so does humanity as a whole adopt crippling methods for achieving security. Both show the infantile compulsive behavior of arrested development. And both can and will be altered.

9. Body and Mind

The ability for individual adjustment increases gradually as we pass from the lowest forms of life to the top of the tree of evolution. The nervous system increases accordingly in complexity, from a rudimentary excitability to the creative mind. Parallel to this increasing complexity of the nervous function, we see an increasing ability for active change and for molding the environment to fit individual requirements. The lower forms of life either perish or thrive according to whether the prevalent conditions fit them or not. For every spore, plant, or bacteria that survives, millions perish. In the highest animal we find the greatest ability for individual adjustment, the greatest variety of individual requirements, and consequently the most active transformation of the environment to meet each individual's needs. Finally, note that speech, the use of hands, erect posture, and all the other human features are to be found in rudimentary forms in many other animals. But in no other species is there such a variety of differences between one individual and the other as in men.

To explain this differentiation, numerous devices have been invented: luck, a soul capable of reincarnation that bears the marks of consecutive lives, an unconscious that has a life of its own and that has its own way, probability, and inherent intelligence. All these and other devices have had this in common—they have ascribed individual traits of behavior to something *beyond our influence,* that is, something outside and independent of the material support, so that we believe that we are not really responsible for behaving as we do. Heretofore there was also little scope for changing or otherwise influencing the human frame in a manner more fitting to the demands we make on it. The only thing left to do was to be good, to appease the gods, repent, expiate, confess, be analyzed—all more or less a passive surrendering dictated by impotence, guilt, or shame. If nothing happened, at least the fault was with (as the Bible says) our ancestors whose sins linger unto the fourth generation.

With increasing knowledge and greater ability to bring about changes in the environment and in our own bodies, a more potent and mature attitude becomes possible. The essential difficulties are largely unsolved, but it is time to relinquish our passive attitude.

These difficulties are not as great as they seem if we remember that all human brains are not identical. Anatomy, physiology, psychology, and other sciences studying the human organism have hitherto examined the similarities between different individuals and thus produced a nucleus of reliable facts that enable us to understand those functions of our bodies that are common to all of us. It was found that what is common to men is also common to other animals, and we have had to accept the idea that we are not much different from them. But in our present state of knowledge we can now also see that the human nervous system has some features that account for the individual differences in us and that at the same time explain the essential differentiation between men and other animals. In the final analysis, the ability of the human nervous system to make individual patterns, or the ability to learn from personal experience, is so much greater in man that we can consider it as a new quality.

Most of the difficulties we encounter in understanding ourselves are due to considering adult functioning and behavior as intrinsic human qualities and forgetting that the history of the individual is indissoluble from him. We tend to believe that we come to the world with a preset pattern or ensemble of characteristics and that we would be what we are now even if our history were not what it was. Inadvertently we continue to consider life as a series of static states in which we find ourselves and not as a process. Most of us conceive the relationship between the environment and men as similar to that which exists between the elements and a stone. A stone has its identity, and the elements can change the shape and state of vitrification, but it remains essentially the same stone, with few individual differences from other bits of the same stone.

In the human being, however, the nervous system is so affected during the prolonged childhood by its personal experience of the environment that it grows into a being with personal characteristic reactions, biological as well as emotional, that are unique for each personal experience.

A human offspring having grown up in a matriarchal society is quite a different human being and has quite distinct characteristics from one raised in a patriarchal society. A savage is different from a civilized man and the essential difference is what happened to them after birth. Ignoring the greater importance of personal experience and its effects on the human nervous system one instant and forgetting inheritance in the next, we find ourselves agreeing with such statements as the following:

The greatness or the smallness of a man is determined for him at his birth, as strictly as it is determined for a fruit, whether it is to be a currant or an apricot. Education, favorable circumstances, resolution, industry, may do much, in a certain sense they do *everything;* that is to say, they determine whether the poor apricot shall fall in the form of a green bead, blighted by the east wind, and be trodden under the foot; or whether it shall expand into tender pride and sweet brightness of golden velvet.*

without being shocked by their contradictions.

Our ideas of human nature, character, and action are a collection of contradictory half-truths, held together by a thin veneer of beautiful but empty phraseology. There is no doubt that at conception it is very strictly determined whether the newborn offspring is going to be a human being or an apricot. Thereafter, favorable circumstances, resolution, and industry have, if we know how to use them, at least as much importance as our inheritance, provided we have normal human structure. But no amount of industry or resolution on the part of an apricot will make the slightest difference to its greatness or golden-velvety appearance for that matter, only favorable circumstances are necessary. Passive, vegetative reliance on circumstances as a means of subsistence is a condition met with only in children or in immature

---

*John Ruskin, *Modern Painters,* Chapter III, p. 44.

people with arrested development and fixed infantile reactions. Circumstances in men are actively arranged, collectively and individually, to fit their state and their means. Only a few elementary things are predetermined, and those that are strictly predetermined—such as the color of the eyes, the texture of the skin or similar attributes—are of secondary importance most of the time and very rarely affect the greatness or smallness of a man.

Without a guiding principle, it is obviously not easy to correlate the facts that we observe. On the one hand, we often see people preserving certain modes of behavior, practically unchanged, notwithstanding the hardest shocks that life may give them. Calamities and luck are taken in stride, and the person seems to remain or even become more his old self. The easiest explanation of permanence of character "inherited" from ancestors suggests itself at once. On the other hand, we see social position, wealth, and opportunity making such an enormous difference, and so radically altering the behavior of many individuals, that we are equally convinced that circumstances are the only things that really matter. The confusion is due largely to our forgetting that our logical thinking deals of necessity with abstractions and to our also forgetting that we have not considered reality, but only a simplification of it.

In fact, there is not a single case of a child, having had its character analyzed and recorded at birth, who was maintained in a strictly unchanging enviroinment so that the "inherited" characteristics, such as possessiveness, sense of justice, and parental love, could be compared to those of other people. All our opinions on the innate properties of the human frame, on their constancy or malleability in the face of environmental change, are based on the analysis of behavior in which the factors of a human body and an environment have already very intricately affected each other. Thus we extrapolate, guess, and base our opinions on what are only more or less plausible assertions.

Even simply imagining experiments and following them through in our imagination would produce better conclusions, provided we keep our convictions in abeyance while imagining.

Thus, in the above mentioned imaginary experiment we are forced to admit that we cannot determine the character of a newborn baby, even if we *could* actually experiment with it. Not a single trait of behavior can be established with any probability at all without taking into account the environment and circumstances such as the properties of the parents, their social status, and the baby's place in the family. But all this information is so scanty that anybody's guess is as good as anybody else's. In fact we are forced to admit that we cannot know the innate propensities before there is a considerable interaction between them and the environment. In other words, character has no meaning without environment. We form an idea of a person's character when we know how he behaves in given conditions, and how consistently he repeats himself in the same circumstances. We cannot speak sensibly of character without taking into consideration the personal experience of the individual—a fact that we keep forgetting most of the time. Character is a preferred pattern of behavior, formed by each individual through personal experience of the environment. It is important to find out what are the significant factors in personal experience that produce individual differences. What are the parts of our system that are affected in such a way that our future reactions become more predictable? And how does all this happen? We are thus brought to the problem of body-mind relationship and especially to that part of it that differs markedly from individual to individual.

In ancient Greece and Rome, it was believed that the heart was the seat of goodness or wickedness, the spleen the seat of temper, the loins the seat of strength, and (Aristotle) that the power of reason resided in the brain. On the whole, the human body was an instrument through which universal qualities manifested themselves if they chose to do so. To think differently from others, one had to be inspired. If the thought was good, one was possessed by a good spirit. If it was bad, one was possessed by an evil spirit. It was thought that immaterial essence becomes imprisoned in the body, mostly for the purpose of purifying it through suffering. The "I" had "free will," which could either lead to the salvation of the soul and raise it to higher levels, or degrade it and cause its perdition.

Today we believe that the nervous system is the seat of both emotive and reasoning phenomena. But somehow even now we cannot really accept that some gray matter in the nervous system could have that much to do with "spiritual" and "noble" qualities. We halfheartedly reject the old ideas and replace them by others that are not less nebulous than the old, such as *mind, will,* and *the unconscious.* I say "nebulous," not because there are no manifestations that justify such classifications, but because we are apt to forget that these are classification terms and thus read into them existence per se.

Mind, the unconscious, and will, have no more existence than velocity. There is no velocity without matter, although we can speak of "change of velocity" and call it acceleration. Mind, the unconscious, and will are functions; they have no existence before action has taken place. They describe a relationship mode of action and nothing else. This problem is perhaps the most controversial of all problems in history, and it would be more than presumptuous to think that we have said the last word on it. I believe, however, that this present evaluation is worthwhile, as it suggests action where before it seemed as if there were nothing we could do.

Speech, the use of hands, erect carriage, active modification of the environment to fit biological properties, the ability of individual adjustment as distinct from species adaptation to environment, and many additional features distinguish men from other animals. All these qualities are not fundamentally human; they can be found in rudimentary forms, separately or in groups, in other animals. There is little doubt that the nervous system plays a greater part than any other part of the body in these phenomena. First, we will make ourselves a picture of the workings of the human nervous system and then of the role played by the body in our mental makeup.

The nervous system consists of matter contained in the cavity of the cranium and that of the spinal cord, the nerves, and some nervous masses (or ganglia) in front of the spine, called the *auto-*

nomic or *vegetative nervous system.* Most of the nervous system consists of white matter, but the outer layers of the brain are grey. These outer layers form the rind, or the *cortex,* of the brain. Certain areas of the cortex are concerned with activating the muscles; they form the *motor cortex.* Other areas are concerned with appreciation of impulses arriving from the senses; they form the *sensory areas.*

The number of cells in the brain is remarkably constant for each species. These cells do not divide continuously like other cells; they all cease multiplying in the first months after birth, and most of them stop dividing *long* before that. The difference in weight between the adult and the newborn brain is due to the growth of the cells, and especially the growth of their ramifications. The basic structure and number of the cells of the nervous system, however, are the same throughout the whole lifetime of the individual.

Every function necessitates the coordinated activity of numerous cells. The connections, or paths, between the cells cooperating for all those actions or functions that are essential to life must therefore be ready at birth. In this category, we find breathing, swallowing, digestion, and excretion—in short, all the purely vegetative acts. The command of the skeletal muscles, for voluntary acts, is very rudimentary at birth. A special bundle of nervous cells and fibers called the *pyramidal tract* must grow down into the spinal cord before impulses from the cortical motor areas can reach the spinal nerves, which alone have direct connections with the skeletal muscles. No skeletal muscle is directly connected to the cortex. Long before voluntary movements are possible, the body responds by reflex contractions only. In these reflex acts, the higher nervous centers generally take no positive, active part, although their inhibitory effect is frequent.

It is important to bear in mind that we have only one means of action, namely muscular contraction, and that there is a whole series of sources of nervous impulses commanding these muscles. The lowest centers produce purely reflective contractions; the centers above may enhance or inhibit the lower impulses; the centers higher still may lift the inhibition of the center immediately below and enhance the lowest source, or vice versa. The highest centers are most active during the process of forming new responses or when inhibiting habitual or automatic acts.

There are definite sensory areas on the surface of the brain for visual, auditory, taste, and other sensations. Around each area is a larger area in which memories or associations connected with the senses are stored. In some parts of the brain, "localization" is extremely precise. Thus, the retina, for instance, has a point-for-point projection on the visual area at the back of the brain. Every perception is a composite phenomenon involving separate senses and various parts of the body, so that the memory of it is fixed in many different parts of the brain. Injury to particular areas often produces quite amazing results. Thus, there are persons who cannot write numbers but are able to write certain dates; others who cannot write a certain letter of the alphabet, but find no difficulty in writing the words containing it.

Localization in the brain is functional. The association area for recognizing writing is in the visual area, while that for spoken words is in the auditory area. Recollection of written words is in the area concerned with the muscular control of the fingers as well as those other parts of the body that cooperate in the act of writing.

It must be understood that the cortical motor area does not have an executive function; instead, it facilitates the motor impulses or incitements that are produced under the influence of other nervous centers, or in response to irritations from the body and its environment. The cortex sends impulses to the lower motor centers in the spine, which (among others) execute the muscular contractions necessary to perform movement. The muscles are not entirely inert; they are usually in a state of tonic contraction at the moment of receiving any motor impulse. The tonic contraction is due to the response of the lower centers to the gravitational forces acting on the different segments of the body and the viscera. Any voluntary movement means, therefore, an enhancement of the contraction of some muscles and a decontraction of their antagonists; that is, those muscles that produce diametrically opposed effects. Each articulation is provided with sets of muscles having the opposite effect on it.

The extent of the motor cortical areas not only corresponds to the size or bulk of the organs but also to function. Thus, the area concerned with the thumb is considerably larger than the area concerned with the leg. An important particularity of the human cortex consists in that no two human adult brains are exactly alike. Exciting similar spots in two different brains does not produce the same effects; somehow the history of individual experience is written into the cortex. Whether the excitation of a given point will contract or decontract a given muscle depends not only on general localization, but also on what happened to that muscle before. There are no such pronounced individual differences in other animals.

This is a point of capital importance: *the anatomy of the human brain is affected by individual history to a degree unknown in other animals.* To my mind, the elucidation of this particularity sheds a light by which the body-mind relationship can be better understood, and a new approach to many difficult problems illuminated. The human brain differs from those of other animals in many additional respects, but those other differences are *gradual* along the ladder of evolution. There is no sudden jump sufficiently significant that wholly accounts for the observed differences in their behavior. However, a sharp difference between the brains of men and other animals is found if we divide the weight of the adult brain by the weight of the brain at birth. In man the weight differential is about 5, rarely going up to 7. In the anthropoid ape, it is about 1.5, and in most lower mammals even nearer to 1.

The nervous system gradually evolves from the outer envelope of the embryo and structurally resembles the skin cells. Besides the inner activity of the higher nervous centers and the regulation of body processes, the nervous system deals mainly with two things: (1) the conduction of information both from outside of the body and from the muscles, tendons, and ligaments, toward the center, and (2) the issuing and conveying of motor impulses to the muscles. The body itself may be considered as part of the environ-ment of the nervous system, so that the autonomic nervous system that deals with the vegetative processes of the body, and mainly helps to adjust it to rapid changes, also falls into the preceding categories.

All manifestation of life is expressed through movement, and nervous activity, except for maintaining the body in a state en-abling it to act, is therefore concerned mostly with displacing masses; that is, with antigravitational adjustment. Although we often do not think of the fact that life and movement are practi-cally the same thing, we do nevertheless make our fundamental classification of the living world after the mode of gravitational adaptation. Thus we speak of *reptiles, fish, birds,* and *animals,* mean-ing "crawling," "swimming," "flying," and "walking": all differ-ent ways of moving in spite of gravitation. It is not surprising, therefore, that movement (or action in general) would be an essen-tial characteristic of any individual nervous system. We have seen that the adult human brain is unique and, in fact, we can differen-tiate quite readily between individuals by their simplest attitudes and movements. The posture and movements of other animals, birds, fish, or reptiles are incomparably less individual. Therefore, paradoxical as it may seem at first, the human mind depends more on the history of its body than is the case with other living beings. For instance, the cortical mechanisms concerned with speech are a genetic inheritance. Although the experiment has never been made, to my knowledge, a human baby isolated from all contact from the instant of birth would nevertheless have very probably a much richer and varied vocal command and expression than any other animal. Yet it would speak no language and its mental capac-ity would be greatly reduced accordingly.*

A dog raised in isolation from birth, however, does not differ very materially from any other dog in respect to its vocal abilities.

---

*There is somewhere in the Talmud an account of a king who made such an experiment in order to find out what is the natural language of men. And as the story goes, the first word the boy said when brought among men, was the Hebrew word for "bread." No comment.

The individual experience in men is of greater consequence because the growth of the brain after birth is so considerable (5 to 7 times). From this example and from what we have said before, we are led to think that the part of the brain that is so influenced by the actual experience of the individual consists of the paths and connections between the cortical motor and association cells, depending on cell processes and their ramifications. Evidence in support of this is found in the fact that all functions that need no apprenticeship (such as breathing) or those that need very little (such as swallowing, digestion, and other vegetative processes) are ready to function at the same time as in other animals, and the individual differences, if any, are insignificant.

In general, the longer the infancy period of a living being the greater is the capacity for individual adjustment; that is, the ability to modify the response to fit the environment. The more an animal is fit to look after itself as soon as it is born, the less it is capable of learning. Obviously, in such cases, the paths and nervous interconnections must be ready made. Herd animals, for instance, are born with all the paths of the nervous system completely formed, so that the newborn can follow the herd at once. All animals that we refer to as calves are in this category. The mountain animals, goats, and the like are equally capable of moving about soon after birth. All these infants can not only walk, run, and jump but can also right themselves when falling or skidding. Their adjustment to changing environmental contours is almost as perfect as in the adult, and their nervous mechanisms must therefore be in the same state. They need not, and practically cannot, learn any new individual actions. The motor incitement sources of impulses, and the muscles, are connected in preset precise patterns of action. To learn a new act is a long and difficult job; the inborn pattern must be undone and a new one formed. This rarely happens spontaneously. Only in artificial conditions requiring much knowledge and experience is it possible to teach such animals some new tricks, and it is essential to start very early, before the short childhood is over. The growth of the nervous system is minimal, and there is little room for individual adjustment.

In contrast, the human child has most of his functions approximately in the same state as that of speech; that is, the executive muscles are under the influence of the lower nervous centers and respond reflectively in a few elementary patterns. Therefore, the crying of most babies is largely indistinguishable one from another. Only expert observers can tell the cry of one from the other, just as it requires an expert tracker with long experience to tell the difference in hoofprints from one horse to another. The striking vocal distinctions that enable the lowest intelligence to tell one adult human voice from another at a great distance are lacking.

In the same way all the skeletal muscles can respond reflectively; the reaction to falling, for instance, can be elicited within a few minutes after birth, even though no accomplished act comparable to that of a day-old calf's motion is possible for several years. In the human being, the individual experience of the environment sets the paths and forms the connections of the motor cortical patterns, while in other animals they are mostly preset and innate. The preset patterns of other animals may be considered as the experience of the species, and the mode of reaction is instinctive. The instinctive response fits conditions similar to those in which the ancestral learning took place and has a great biological economy. In man, instinctive behavior is much less important. In human society, stereotyped ancestral responses are rarely fitting, because there are only few situations that call for identical responses from all of us. Only in very elementary acts, and those concerned with preservations of organs from violent injury, can we find instinctive elements in our actions. The nervous paths and patterns are formed under the influence of the environment, and the final act is the result of individual experience and inheritance.

A mental picture of the working of the nervous and muscular mechanisms might be helpful here in understanding some aspects of the problem. But the reader must use careful judgment to counteract the tendency to describe as identical, because of their partial similarities, the processes under examination and the analogy. The motor cells of the cortex may be thought of as batteries, the motor nerves as wire leads, and the muscles as tiny motors. In the human infant there is practically no connection between the batteries and the motors as far as voluntary movements go. The association bundles—particularly the pyramidal tract that joins the motor cortex to the spinal cord—take a long time to grow. These bundles are very rudimentary at birth, growing rapidly at first and continuing to grow up to the age of twenty-two or -three. We can imagine, therefore, that in animals the leads are permanently connected to the batteries at birth or practically so, while in men these connections are made under the influence of personal experience. For dissimilar acts, different kinds of connections will be established according to (1) the permanency and (2) the identical recurrence of the situations requiring these acts.

In every act, only some of the motor cells of the cortex are actively involved, while the others must be inhibited. Thus, we can (very roughly) imagine a switchboard with plug holes, one for each battery, and a series of plugs to which the wire leads from the muscles are connected for each action. In the human being, as far as the voluntary acts are concerned, these plugs are made up in accordance with each individual's personal experience of the environment. But before we indulge in our analogy, an important point must be made. Every muscle can be contracted in two separate ways—tonically and voluntarily. These contractions differ in many ways. The tonic contraction is slower and can be maintained for very long periods of time with little muscular or nerve fatigue. The term *fatigue* must be understood here to mean the ability to reproduce the same action when the same impulses flow through the nerves to reach the muscles, and not the feeling of tiredness. The tonic contraction is due mostly to the red fibers of the muscles while the voluntary contractions involve the white fibers, which contract faster and more powerfully but fatigue much sooner. The impulses producing the tonic contractions come from the lower centers of the nervous system, while the impulses producing voluntary contractions come from the motor cortex or are initiated by it.

The tonic contraction of the muscles of the body is the result of the species adaptation to the forces of gravitation and is an innate property of the nervous system of each species. For example, the jaw is lifted and the mouth closed without our doing or thinking anything whatsoever. The weight of the jaw pulls on it, and this pull activates the proprioceptive nerve fibers in the muscles of the jaw to send impulses that cause a contraction just sufficient to lift the jaw into its habitual position. The jaw never drops down, even though our head remains in the vertical position for days on end. In the jaw, the voluntary contraction is superimposed onto the tonic contraction. Thus we can also open the jaw; that is, the voluntary impulses can decrease or increase the state of contraction of each skeletal muscle, every one of which contains a sufficient number of white fibers for controlling voluntary movement. (To be really precise, we would have to complicate the picture, for indirectly we can also contract the involuntary muscles. We will describe one important means of doing so later on.)

To return to our analogy—among the immense numbers of combinations possible, some groups of batteries are used most of the time. In these instances, there is an advantage in having the connections permanent, so the wire leads are soldered onto the batteries. This sort of thing illustrates true reflex action.

Somewhat greater freedom in altering connections is found in the patterns that are used continuously, but with occasional switchovers to other patterns. The heartbeat, breathing, and the like are representative of this kind of connection. In specifically human actions (such as speech, erect carriage, conscious thought, piano playing, mathematics, or other creative activities), there are no connections that are in working condition at birth; there is only the *tendency* to proceed with the activity that forms them. The actual pattern of connections of motor and association centers to their subcortical ganglia and bundles depends on the time in which the individual lives and the social group and environment in which he grows up. Had these patterns been preset, our thinking, language, music, and mathematics would be as similar to those of the fathers of the human race as our breathing, swallowing, and other vegetative functions still are.

For the specifically human acts, we may think of the leads or wires to the executive organs as connected to multiple-pin plugs. The environment and personal experience fixes the individual wires to the pins, and the voluntary act plugs the plug onto the switchboard. This unique human capacity for adjustment corresponds to the great number of path combinations possible, and the ability to learn corresponds to the freedom of making individual patterns. In actions that change from instance to instance, the permanency of the connections is only slight. In others they may be compared to leads held by nuts screwed on with degrees that range from finger tight to dead tight.

If we could "see" the natal cortex of a calf or a kid, we would find that the connections of the cells concerned with walking (whether the calf has walked or not), as well as the leads going to the spinal nerves, are all "wired up." In a human brain, we would find practically no connections for voluntary walking, the "wiring" being formed according to individual trial-and-error experience, with some connections being made and then undone to form a better pattern or simply falling into disuse. The experience of the body is, therefore, of special importance in men as it forms the nervous mechanisms that arrange and direct the ulterior experience of the body.

This analogy, or mental picture, gives a clearer insight into the working of our mind and body in many instances where it remains obscure and unintelligible. The congenitally blind, for instance, express anger and fear as other people do when the outburst is spontaneous, but they cannot reproduce the necessary mimicry to order. The visual experience seems to be indispensable for the ability to do so. The voluntary innervation has grown without the visual experience, and the motor pattern in question has never been formed.

The patterns for standing, sitting, and speaking are literally the product of the age in which we live, the social group into which we are born, and in general our individual experience.

The freedom of making up nervous connections as a consequence of each individual history implies at the same time lesser stability in these patterns. They are more temporary and easier to change than the congenitally preset ones. Setting about it the right way, we can alter the cortical patterns from English to Hindustani, or the other way around. The same is true of all the other human functions that were formed through our personal experience, such as walking, sitting, thinking, or any other act of doing that has necessitated personal apprenticeship. Individual experience in man is part of his physiological process of maturing, and human nature is the most flexible, temporary, and adjustable nature of all. Only ignorance can fully account for the apparent fixity or permanency of some features of human behavior. As long as we continue forming traditional responses in the growing nervous system, we are bound to find what we should expect, namely the resulting traditional examples. With scanty knowledge of reality of which our nervous mechanism is such a very important part, tradition (imperfect as it is) cannot be thrown away lightheartedly. But it is also time to realize that our shortcomings are the result of our refusal to take responsibility for our ignorance. Like children, we prefer to shift responsibility onto Adam and Eve and original sin, instead of having to do something about setting things right. In general, instilling stereotyped behavior in the higher mental activities is literally acting against natural tendencies, as we thereby throw away the most properly human property of the nervous system.

In respect to the *higher* human functions, the brain is a blank that is filled in by the intermediary of the sensory and motor body experience. One who is congenitally deaf has no personal experience of language, forms no cortical motor patterns for using the vocal apparatus, and can never speak a single word, although the nervous and muscular elements involved are perfectly normal. The argument for the importance of the body experience in forming the paths and patterns of our brain becomes even more convincing when we know that once the body experience has taken place and some connections for definite patterns have been made, a person may well become totally deaf without materially affecting the ability to speak. The brain itself makes no connections for any of the specifically human functions and, unlike other land mammals, makes no definite standing pattern. Although I have no experimental evidence for it, I do believe that a baby with congenital blindness kept in total immobility on its back until the pyramidal tract has more or less completely grown (which takes approximately twenty-three years) would never spontaneously adopt a truly erect human posture. But a calf in an equivalent experiment would quickly adopt a true bovine carriage.

The body and mind relationship can now be understood more clearly. At birth only the vegetative system and the part of the brain concerned with reflex movements are more or less in working condition. The paths and patterns of the higher functions have yet to be formed: for this, a prolonged use of the muscles and at least some use of the senses is essential. Once these connections and paths have been formed, the material envelope of the soma becomes less and less essential. When the brain has reached maturity, its functioning is practically independent of any particular muscular group or sense. Only in the elementary, strictly localized functions of the part of the body involved will any deficiencies be found. The paths and patterns, once formed, carry around in them the complete memory of all perceptions, sensations, and actions. The brain is now capable of forming new patterns by regrouping the existing ones; that is, it is capable of thinking, imagining, and inventing.

Thus, the loss of an arm in an adult does not eliminate its participation in mental functions. In coordinating his movements, he will behave as if the arm were still there, so that he will not stand any nearer than before to a table placed on the side of the missing arm. The cortical pattern has been formed thanks to the influence of the arm and remains active.

This unique property of the human nervous system—its capacity for forming nervous paths through individual experience—of necessity entails less permanency of these paths than of the innate ones, and thereby implies greater facility for regroupment into new patterns. Hence the human facility to modify response to stimuli; that is, to learn. The ability to think and imagine is innate, but the actual thoughts, as well as the content or material of dreams and imaginings, are the product of individual experience. They are similar in similar social groups, and nations, in which the individual experiences are sufficiently stereotyped. The elements of thoughts, dreams, and other mental manifestations are extremely diverse in individuals belonging to widely differing social groups; for instance, between a Zulu and a European surrealist painter. In short, the use and experience of the body are necessary in order to form the mental functions. After the formation of a sufficient number of paths and patterns, the somatic support becomes less and less essential; we can think—that is, reexcite the formed patterns, regrouping them into new ones. This common experience of the gradual liberation of the cerebral functions from the somatic support, although perhaps not so clearly formulated, may have provided the clue for the idea of a soul or a mind altogether free from material support. We must beware of falling into a similar trap; we must not imagine that such liberation really occurs. It does not. In practice, the state of the envelope of the nervous system is of paramount importance. The functioning of the higher nervous centers is extremely sensitive to what happens to the body for the simple reason that there is no separate existence of these parts in a living individual. How great this interdependence is, and to what extent the one can be affected through the other, are the main subjects of the following chapters.

A CLEARER PICTURE

The baby's environment, in the shape of the parents, is moved by the emotional stresses set up in them. In the most general form, if viewed from the baby's standpoint, these stresses come under the heading of the dependence relationship. The environment can and does act on the baby by direct manipulation of the body. For a comparatively long time, there is no alternate way of influencing the brain and the nervous mechanisms by any other means than observable physical changes produced in the immediate vicinity of the envelope of the nervous system, which is, most significantly, the new identity.

The human nervous system has some similarities to those of other animals, but differs from them in many respects. The most important difference consists in the lack of connections between the motor areas of the cortex, and the musculature. A comparatively long time will pass before the nervous tracts bridging the gap between the motor centers and the muscular system will make the first significant step on the road of destroying the utter dependence of the baby on his parents.

Because of this peculiarity of the human nervous system, there are practically no innate, well-formed patterns of response, as found in other animals. Thus all analogies from animal behavior do not apply to men without careful qualifications. Very grave mistakes causing much personal misery are due to the unqualified acceptance of both the innate theory and the theory of animal behavior as a guide to correct human behavior, especially in the sexual plane.

The living body is endowed with periodic activities. Breathing, food intake, sexual activity, waking and sleeping, action and rest are all produced by periodic changes that grow to a climax of tension to be released by the external environment. Every animal has to find itself an environment that provides the means for the adequate release of these tensions. Most animals have their nervous systems more fully developed in a very short time after birth; the human nervous system matures during a very long period after birth. The means for releasing the periodic climaxes of tension are therefore more dependent on the environment in man than in any other living species. A human shows very weak tendencies for relieving these tensions in a specific way. His food intake depends almost exclusively on the habits he has formed, and as these take a long time they remain plastic and can be molded very easily. In the faster-growing animals, habits become set much more readily and are more fixed. The same is true of all the other tensions and their modes of release.

A detailed and illuminating study of the stability or instability of human "instincts" as compared with animals can still be found in Metchnikoff's *The Nature of Man* (a rather old book, but a very good one nevertheless). Metchnikoff shows quite convincingly that we commit a fundamental and very grave mistake by assuming that human behavior is controlled to a considerable extent by innate "instincts."

In short, we may take it as a correct first approximation that human behavior is mostly directed by the habits formed in each individual in the world of his own personal experience. The Arab male, for instance, remains largely indifferent to the sight of female breasts; European males are sexually inhibited by a woman smelling of rancid butter, while men of some African tribes are very much excited by it; and so on. Human sexual behavior is as much a product of the environment, and the social order for the civilized man, as are his food habits.

We can imagine that if the dependence relationship were of constant intensity and direction, without very violent variations, the food habits, sexual habits, and all the other habits of thought and action would develop in one direction and would foster a nonconflicting mode of response in the individual. But such an individual would have little plasticity; he would be in all respects like the dog who must continue chasing the cat. Once such a habit has been allowed to form, his behavior would be stereotyped and predictable.

A human being with a relatively sheltered and uneventful emotional past would have little capacity to cope with rapidly changing emotional stresses. He would therefore shun such situations and would form a conservative attitude to life. People in remote rural districts show in fact a greater tendency to conservatism. Were it not for the imagination fostered by fairy tales in early infancy and by schooling later on, most people would be even more conservative than they are.

Thanks to imagination, no child has an absolutely uneventful emotional life, even when it is intentionally sheltered from disturbances. I remember being taken to a small village in early childhood where I saw a pig being killed for Christmas. The gory sight and the screams of the animal made an indelible impression on me. I imagined myself tied up and helpless in the hands of adults, who could, after all, do the same thing to me if they decided to do so. I can now see quite clearly how my previous experience led to great sensitivity on this plane and how subsequent events confirmed me in my apprehension. I had to become strong and always be ready. And only later, on reaching a Black Belt standard in judo, did I to a certain measure work out the kink in me due to that unfortunate experience. I cite this example to show that strong emotional upheavals often take place in very quiet surroundings and in apparently quite ordinary circumstances. Thus, thanks to imagination two twins who are living a seemingly identical life may have quite different behavior patterns. However, an argument is usually brought forth, because of the external similarities of the twins, in support of the view that behavior is inherited, and that in spite of identical conditions people behave according to their innate character.

The utter dependence of the child on his parents during a prolonged period of time is responsible for the fact that almost hermetically sealed compartments of given sets of behavior are formed, and it is left to the internal processes to resolve the contradictions. The child is taught to speak the "absolute" truth, but he soon finds that the parents themselves do not abide by this rule. He thus learns, by reality-testing, the importance of expediency. In our society a child has very little chance of being able to test the absolute and often quite erroneous social ideas held about sex, and about human behavior in general. A considerable number of people, therefore, grow up with crude notions on the subject, and find it extremely difficult to resolve the conflict that is bound to arise in the face of reality.

The earliest interaction of the child with the external world is entirely physical. The earliest emotional movements become, therefore, associated or linked with muscular and postural patterns. The emotions are thus reinstated when there is sufficient resemblance or contrast between the present body state and the original one. By and by with the multiplication of experience, the origin becomes less and less distinct. Our anger, for example, often begins long before it is externalized. In that case we become aware of the body state associated with anger in our personal experience. We can learn to become aware of that state in time, and to check it.

Because every one of us is aware of when this happens in ourselves, we cannot understand neurotic people who seem to be unable to check themselves. We, therefore, frequently believe they do not try or do not really want to do so. We often hear the exhortation "pull yourself together." Does anyone really know how one pulls oneself together? It is the crux of the problem. The neurotic certainly makes an effort, but he pulls himself to pieces instead of pulling himself together. He believes he strives to do the right thing while doing the wrong one. The same is true in those cases of an inability to achieve positive action where the exhortation is "pull yourself up." The attempts to do so are not much different from pulling oneself together.

What is needed is a positive method of directing oneself, a way whereby one can learn to produce the wanted effect without, at the same time, bringing on unwanted impulses—in short, the physiology of "doing."

Habitual patterns are reinstated by abstract mental associations, by vegetative states of the body, by muscular and attitudinal patterns, all formed, in a most personal manner, in the course of one's personal history. Analysis has taught us the structure and the material out of which our personality is built up. But for the synthesis of the new personality to emerge from the debris of the old one we rely on something to "click" in the person's mind.

Without teaching a better method of self-direction, one finds oneself perforce using the old habitual way, recreating or placing oneself in conditions with which one can deal, even though they are painful. Therefore, on top of the mental rejection of the old habit, a vegetative distaste and body discomfort must be created with the unwanted pattern. And, what is more important still, a new set of habits must be cultivated methodically from the start, so that the discarded ones need not be reinstated, as they otherwise inevitably will be.

This reinstatement of the old habit is general, and acting against it is sensed as "resistance." The person knows that he is wrong, but—having no substitute for the habitual use—he can hardly do anything else except retire into himself and do nothing at all or "resist." The length of the treatment and the imperfect results are due to want of synthetic action, the lack of positive means of doing better than before.

The reinstatement of the old habits is due to the fact that habits, bad or good, yield results and are therefore sustained by the environment. They could be built up if they never yielded any results at all. The only thing that makes them wrong is that they do not release the tension that moves us to action in a satisfactory manner, so that the tension continues to urge us into activity—into repetition of the same action, with the same result, and so on until exhaustion.

10. Action, Inhibition, and Fatigue

All action of a living being is accomplished through muscular contraction or release. The voluntary control of muscles in human beings is acquired through long and laborious experience. In the fetus, any excitation spreads indiscriminately all over the musculature. In adulthood, when we attempt a new action we find a similar but less pronounced spreading of contraction. Thus, if we try to skate, ride a bicycle, type, swim, or learn any new skill, we find our muscles enacting not only the projected act but also much else that is unnecessary and often contradictory to the motivated action.

Learning to inhibit unwanted contractions of muscles that function without, or in spite of, our will, is the main task in coordinating action. We have to learn to inhibit those cells of the motor cortex to which the excitation spreads. Before we become able to excite a precise pattern of cells in the wanted order, the neighboring cells all along the pattern of the cells essential to the movement become active. After adequate apprenticeship, when proficiency is achieved, only those cells that command the muscles for the desired performance alone send out impulses. All the others are inhibited. Without this inhibition, no coordinated action is possible.

The sensation of difficulty or resistance to action is indirectly due to imperfect inhibition of the cells commanding the antagonists of muscles that are indispensable in forming the desired pattern. Most of the time it is not the simple inability to inhibit the parasitic contractions that is the problem, but the attempt to simultaneously enact mutually exclusive patterns. When there is real lack of contraction power in that the resistance is not due to imperfect inhibition of the unwanted parasitic contractions (as when we try to push a cathedral), no movement or displacement actually takes place. Correct coordinated action seems, and feels, effortless no matter how great the actual amount of work involved may be. This assertion may seem sweeping, but it can be shown to be true in every case. It suffices to watch the skillful performance of masters in their trades or arts to become convinced that the presence of effort is the indication of imperfect action.

A motor cell or a small number of cells when called on to produce intense excitation, while the adjacent cells are inhibited, fatigues after a few consecutive repetitions. At the same time, the inhibition of the adjacent cells becomes more laborious and imperfect. Thus when moving one finger in an unaccustomed manner we find that the first few movements correspond well to the intended action, but the following attempts to do so correspond less and less. Parasitic contractions come into action, owing to the spread of excitation to neighboring cells, which thus become activated and the inhibition is removed further afield.

Every one of us has a large number of possible action patterns that have never been used before and that remain therefore entirely foreign. Certain combinations never occur, and a number of cells of the motor cortex may as a result remain dormant, constantly inhibited, or at least rarely active. All the other cells that take part in the more used patterns are repeatedly active. As each cell fatigues rapidly, the frequently used muscles participating in a great variety of acts receive impulses from a large number of different cell groups that control in turn the same muscle. In a woman who has lost her arms and has learned to write with her toes, the leg area of the brain must be larger than usual. Correspondingly, her thumb area is smaller than in other people. When skill is acquired, a considerable number of neighboring cells become capable of arranging themselves in turn in the required pattern of excitation and inhibition, and the act can be repeated an appreciable number of times without loss of perfection.

Motor cells tend to be active on their own accord, at least during the growing period, creating exploratory and investigatory activity at the slightest provocation from the outside world or internal change. New patterns are thus formed, and they tend to repeat themselves. The tendency to repetition is so great that if the environment does not prevent the enactment of the new pattern (by fostering the habitual and therefore preferred other activity or by directly inhibiting the tentative new pattern) it will enact itself at the first opportunity when our vigilance slacks off—during sleep, tiredness, or failing health.

It is worth remembering that dreams are most of the time made up of the material and fragmented patterns of earlier personal experience, which have been at one time in the foreground or in the background of our awareness. Freud, for example, thought that dreams have their origin in the experience of the previous day.

In new acts the excitation of cells is not graded. Only after we have learned to inhibit the cells neighboring those which must be excited, can we grade the intensity of action. The mechanism of gradation of muscular force by contraction of fibers in rotation is not operative in the first stages of learning new acts; in the beginning, we always find excessive muscular tensing and contraction indicating an all-out excitation of many cells. All-out excitation of the motor cells produces fatigue very rapidly. It is known from physiology that the first element to fatigue in a neuromuscular elementary circuit is the motor cell. The junction of the nerve to the muscle—that is, the motor plate ending of the nerve—is the next to fatigue. The muscle itself fatigues last of all, and this happens very rarely.

Normal fatigue of the nervous cells is removed by that spread of inhibition that constitutes sleep. The sensation of tiredness is mostly a cortical phenomenon. In normal and correct activity, the production of waste in the muscles is rarely the first cause of fatigue. Everybody knows from her own experience how rapidly one recovers from normal tiredness if interest or emotions are roused. Inhibition can be removed swiftly, but waste and toxins cannot conceivably be removed in an instant—for this, hours of sleep or rest are normally required.

The first abnormal stage of fatigue in motor cells is the loss of the power of inhibition over them. Fatigued cells keep on producing impulses, resulting in feeble contractions, twitching, and finally complete cramps of the muscles. Disorderly, uncoordinated muscular activity results from the loss of inhibitory control over fatigued motor cells. Without a center of inhibition in the cortex, sleep is impossible. Tired cells form such a center: their excitation subsides, and the inhibition spreads. But fatigued cells keep on sending messages. When cells are seriously strained, we lose our capacity of adequately inhibiting sporadic movement. Even very healthy people, who do not know insomnia, normally cease being able to fall asleep when in a state of violent physical exhaustion.

The initial degrees of fatigue pass off with rest. The question is essentially that of the rest of cortical cells, and not of muscle cells. The latter never fatigue in practice to the extent of not contracting when impulses of normal intensity arrive in the normal way. Thus change is as good as rest. When changing action, we do not necessarily change over to other muscles; only the pattern of cells that issue the impulses to the muscles changes. This is sufficient, as the fatigued cells are not called on to produce excitations, and this alone matters.

In the next stage of fatigue of cortical motor cells, we lose the power of inhibiting whole patterns of complete acts. At this stage we find compulsive mannerisms, such as speaking to ourselves and performing well-coordinated acts, but without intention. It is, however, enough to become aware of this fact, and we are still able to inhibit these actions. The inhibitory control is operative so long as our awareness is not diminished. Here again, the fatigued cells need rest. But conscious inhibition is difficult to maintain for long periods. Therefore, actions that are sufficiently diverse must be used, in order to not excite the fatigued pattern. The new actions must involve another part of the body and a different attitude that will inhibit the fatigued one by physiological processes; that is, the new pattern and the old must be mutually exclusive in function.

Just before complete exhaustion of cells the reinstatement of the fatigued pattern cannot be inhibited any longer by normal means of control, since the power of inhibiting excitation of cells is completely lost. Such extreme cases are outside of this discussion.

In the human cortex, in which there are few ready-made patterns at birth, there is a greater tendency for forming new patterns than in lower animals; hence our greater investigatory curiosity. New patterns are being continuously formed, and there is a strong urge to go on using them. This can be observed in children, who pick up a new word and later on a new form of expression, a new movement of any sort—they keep on repeating the new pattern *ad nauseum* to the exasperation of the impatient adults. This uniquely human tendency to repeat new patterns of action probably has much to do with the normal process of cell fatigue, which lowers the power of inhibiting them. Normally even in children, the succession of repetitions of the newly discovered act is moderate, and the intensity used is equally so. The vegetative processes take their normal course and refit the system for smoother action.

Too prolonged repetition, excessive intensity, and permanent activation of a pattern are the causes of all abnormal fatigue. Even the lower centers producing the tonic contractions of the muscles that extend the articulations in standing can be fatigued in this way and can render these muscles flaccid. It is important to realize that muscles may lack in tone when assuring normal posture and yet produce sufficiently powerful contractions in voluntary acts. The impulses producing tone and those producing voluntary acts are not, as we have already said, of identically the same origin. Even specialists in physical education are not always clear about this distinction, and make the mistake of believing that active exercising of the muscles is all that is needed. They are inclined to blame their pupils and accuse them of lack of cooperation and attention when there is little improvement. But volition only affects the distribution of tone indirectly, and the postural improvement that may occur by simple exercising is due to the right thing being done unwittingly.

Habitually improper posture is not as simple as it may appear to some who think it can be remedied by substituting a better posture for the existing one. In reality, faulty distribution of tone is due to faulty volition in the first place. The conscious control is overriding, and the tonic pattern becomes distorted in the long run. The overworked centers fatigue, and the inhibited ones suffer from dystrophy, and the whole spatial body image is distorted. The body sensation is found unreliable and is compensated for by an increased use of the eyes to supplement and correct the faulty muscular account of the body state in space. A second increased appeal is made to voluntary control and attention. Every action now needs a considerable time of thinking out and preparing for, as can so often be seen in people in that state who are negotiating the steps of the underground or even their own houses.

Constant unwavering attention is difficult to maintain for long periods, hence a permanent sensation of tiredness, irritability, and justified apprehension of failure in all sudden and unpremediated action. (We will return to this problem in due course.)

How does an organism provided with multiple synergetic and overriding controls for self-regulation go out of order? The evasive explanation of predisposition (which is the cause usually advanced for most of us) not only covers up ignorance, but (what is much worse) gives no guidance to any positive action, nor does it even suggest where the necessary knowledge should be sought. Undoubtedly, there are cases where the congenital anatomical deficiency is responsible for the poor adjustment; paradoxically, these are the benign cases, except where the habitual mechanism at work in all of us has also been operating here.

In most cases, deterioration is caused by improper use of self. The word *improper* needs qualification, for my contention is that no person does act wittingly against herself. The use we make of ourselves is the best we can muster with the means at our command at that moment; later we may become aware of other alternatives, but at the moment of action we could not do otherwise. Therefore our use is always the proper one as far as concerns our ability to adjust it at the moment of action. If, say, we stoop badly in walking, it is not because we can do otherwise; but nonetheless, we do make an improper use of the body. *Our use of self is as good as our means at the moment permit.*

We have failed to realize hitherto the role played by individual experience in forming the physiology of our nervous system, and the use we learn to make of ourselves is irrational and haphazard.

We teach such a rigidity of mind and body that we need "breaking in" for any but familiar, habitual conditions. In fact, the human nervous system is eminently suitable for change. Our early experience prepares us for conditions analogous to those known to our parents, allowing only for minor differences. Any significant change demands a deep, revolutionary modification in our attitude and response. Using the property of the nervous system, which we work so hard to diminish, it is possible to form individuals capable of coping with a changing world without such intense emotional upheavals that bring many to prostrated breakdowns.

We find emotional instability almost universally (1) in nations that are in the process of deep social and economic transformation, and (2) in people who dare to deviate from the traditional mode of action of their parents, their class, or social group. Those who have dared to go off the beaten path, and would have had a chance of getting somewhere if they were properly equipped, are precisely those who have failed to make even the usual "success" of their lives.

In our education, we keep on sowing the seed of conflict. All our history is nothing but a long list of "great men" who have in fact gone all wrong by the standards taught us. In spite of all the efforts of their betters and elders to make them think and behave like everybody else, they have nevertheless continued using the essentially human quality of forming, testing, and retesting new patterns of action and thought and have even dared to live by their conclusions. The seed of conflict consists of contradictory patterns being fostered in the young. On one hand, we teach them that to be a Man, one must think for oneself, resist convention, and dare tradition—in other words, "make history," like those who did. On the other hand, the socializing routine to which the young are subjected hammers into them conformity and unquestioning respect for tradition and for the socially accepted. We allow digression from the accepted code only to those who are favored by the gods, who have the "divine spark" in them. But no one can tell divine sparks from ordinary sparks (unless he possesses a divine one himself), and, therefore, one needs encouragement and special circumstances before daring to take to oneself the "right" to consider oneself a creative person. Reluctantly, most people work themselves into snug little corners, to fit their clipped wings. But those who have had the good fortune to come, in time, across a truly human spirit, soon reject stereotyped behavior—and their names are then added to the list of the others who are used to muzzle the next generation. The great majority, however, form the required mental and bodily rigidity, although some of these do not do so quite as wholeheartedly as the rest—they keep on struggling. Among such people we find the great sufferers, with their emotive instability and difficulties of all sort. They rarely have the inclination to follow their parents' professions. They often aspire to belong to a class that is, in some respect or other, above the one in which they were educated. The worst use of self is found among these unconventional people who, at least on one plane of human activity, have not followed the example given to them but have tried new ways and have failed. New paths need not only daring; they also need knowledge. The readiness of the human nervous system to make individual patterns is often a blessing in disguise, because the earlier patterns are more stable than those formed later in life. They need skillful action and knowledge before they can be successfully altered. The earlier patterns are formed under the duress of dependence on society, directly and indirectly, and our behavior therefore has been patterned to follow the beaten path.

During our childhood, we lose a considerable measure of the facility of our nervous system for making individual paths and patterns of action, thanks to parental influence on our immediate environment. The adults foster or exclude what they like. True, most of our experience has stood the test of time, which means that it is possible to exist in such conditions, but such existence is only using a fraction of our potential ability. A large part of the physiological freedom of the human nervous system is circumscribed by social tradition. How much of human possessiveness we owe to our being fed and clothed apart from others, with things that "belong to baby" (of which the adult does not partake because of size), has never been adequately established. The effects that the size of the family and the order of being born into it have on the formation of behavior patterns show how decisive the early environmental influences are in forming the responses that are the nucleus of personality.

Our food habits, sleep, regularity of rest, sex habits, and all the other things we do are all performed by muscular acts. And what is even more significant is that the entire organism must be brought into a state in which it obeys and executes the projected acts. Every muscular voluntary action is associated with a skeletal attitude, a vegetative state of the body with a corresponding emotional background. And, though indirectly, we have significant control over these states, mainly through the voluntary motor centers. But, none of these at first sight intimately and exclusively personal affairs is really divorced from the environment. By its rules of hygiene, parental duties, and all the other traditional legacies of organized life, society produces an environment that molds the growing nervous system more directly than it affects other living things.

Man's potential control of self is virtually absolute, but a lion's share of it is in the hands of men and not in those of the individual. Here we are up against the same complexity we have already encountered, namely, the gradual shifting of importance from the somatic support of the nervous system to the higher integrating centers, which continues and reaches its climax in an ideal and therefore unattainable maturity.

For a clearer understanding of the mechanism of action, it is convenient to divide the entire space into three domains: the outside world, the envelope of the nervous system and its support that is our body, and finally the nervous system itself, where response and action are conceived and produced. There is no action without the three elements together making a unified whole. Only as a matter of convenience may we think of any of them as having an existence separate from the others. Such segregation of the whole generally leads to conclusions that are as remote from reality as most abstractions are.

Thus we are prone to make the mistake of expecting ourselves to act as others do, simply because we ignore for a moment that we cannot isolate a person from her personal experience and her environment without losing something in the process of doing so. Very often where change is needed, the ignored elements are the most important for a correct solution.

Action means change; when the exterior world changes in some detail at least, the body state and configuration also change. The nervous system must be influenced both by the external change and by the body in a way that makes the projected action realizable and inclines us to perform the desired action adequately. We must also constantly keep in mind that in living things we can only speak of *processes* and therefore at any moment we are dealing with instantaneous glimpses, so to speak, of the whole process. If we fail to remember this, we introduce an impression of definiteness into our notions that is never present in reality. For instance, when we say "I want," we may forget that this has little meaning without a prolonged and intricate coexistence of the three components just mentioned. Language is rather a poor tool for describing action, because it is a linear arrangement of ideas following each other, whereas in a process all the elements change together and actually affect each other. Only when we share similar experience of a process do words have real value. They serve then as labels for identifying common sensations.

11. The Aim of Readjustment

We generally consider a person healthy when he has no complaints severe enough to make him seek the advice of a doctor. When he complains of some particular discomfort, the medical practitioner usually diagnoses some sort of illness in an organ or function. The practitioner knows very well that there is no such thing as a diseased liver, heart, or kidney without fairly widespread dysfunctioning in the whole organism. By diagnosing a specific organ as the seat of trouble, the practitioner means that an improvement in the functioning of that organ will relieve most directly the symptoms that brought the patient to him. It has long been realized that this approach to the problem of health is not very satisfactory, as it reduces the general standard of health to a very low level. To reach a better standard, it is necessary to improve housing conditions and food habits, eliminate insecurity, change the monotony of certain professions, and so forth. In short, the environment and our behavior would have to change.

In spite of the shortcomings of medicine in practice, we find the average practitioner's intervention is in fact directed at the very source of the trouble, and in the majority of cases it is all over in a few visits. It is true that before long he will be seeing the patient again, but that is due to the low level of health at which present knowledge and practice maintain us.

When we have to seek the advice of a psychologist, the situation is radically different. Unlike the general practitioner, a psychologist needs an interminable number of consultations before he can see clearly the change point that will produce the most direct results. Obviously his task is more difficult, as the general knowledge of the subject is poor. Nevertheless, a clear definition of the purpose to be achieved should make a very considerable difference. As it is, the purpose of most schools of psychology is to bring the patient to behave as do the majority of people—a very fluid and hazy aim indeed. Concluding that the behavior of the great majority of people is normal behavior, we then believe that of the maladjusted must be due in the final analysis to some constitutional abnormality. On the face of things, this seems a justified conclusion. However, if we try to examine the situation from a more distant point of view, removing ourselves from the situation as far as possible, the continuum of differences between the behavior of the majority of people and that of the maladjusted, which seemed at first so great, can now be seen in a new light. From this distant viewpoint, we can examine the whole process of behavior as a biological universal phenomenon and the normal behavior becomes only a particular sample of human behavior. The normal behavior ceases to be The Human Behavior; that is, a human being left to grow up among wolves or elsewhere would not have the normal human behavior in the same way he would still have human anatomical features.

In short, human behavior is essentially a product of the personal experience of each individual, the sequential nature of the irritations, and their consistency. The human behavior is cultivated, and the differences obtained in different people are not necessarily due to biological normality or abnormality, but to the success or failure of the method of cultivation. This applies to any particular set of patterns that the past history of mankind has led us to accept as normal.

Some people seem to think that a normal person is one who is always happy. Life has little to do with happiness—teeth growing in early childhood is hardly conducive to happiness. Healthy behavior differs from other behavior only in the attitude and the way in which we respond to pleasant or distressful events, regardless of whether we have brought them about or they have happened by themselves. This attitude is the result of the conditional experience of the individual and the way in which he submitted to it. The newborn is submitted to this drill from the very instant he comes into the world through the parents' example or their intended action. In this way the body tensions arising from the physiological processes become linked with acts and situations that will soon feel as natural as the body itself.

At the end of any growth period, the patterns of action and reaction formed during that period demand modification. Weaning, different clothes, changes in toilet training, or changes in mother's attention, are major events. The tendency of all habits is to reproduce themselves. Thus the consistent conditioning of each procedure will show up in the difficulty of introducing any new procedure. Although it may seem that we have done very little to influence the new child one way or the other, we have in fact laid down the foundation and the skeleton of future behavior. The essential patterns are already linked with a certain emotional intensity that will oppose future change. Thus the child may refuse to open his bowels in the new fashion, or may object to the new feeding.

Already he has learned the rudiments of possessiveness in having clothes that nobody puts on but himself, feeding utensils that nobody uses but himself, the small bed that nobody lies on but himself. The difference in size itself, and the civilized habits of men, introduce private possessiveness without the slightest awareness. (A detailed study of the origin of our attitudes along the lines just enumerated is a fascinating affair I hope to deal with elsewhere.) The important thing for us at this junction is that we can already discern "neurotic" and normal behavior. If we did not have to introduce new acts and functions, there would be no greater differences between normal and maladjusted people than the minor differences observed at this age.

As soon as the child learns to speak and walk, very important tendencies are inculcated in the same indirect and unwitting way. By this time, the child has learned that he must be good in order to obtain the affection he needs, and to feel guilty when he is not conforming with the norm of being good laid down by the adult. Eating in order to be big and strong like Daddy and a wealth of other cross motivations are steadily being piled up. Affection is linked, and continues to be linked, with one person of the opposite sex only and so on.

In the next stage of development, most of these patterns will have to be broken up and the emotive drive redirected. The children in whom the formed patterns have not been established with undue repetitiveness and regularity, and without singular emotiveness on the part of the parents, will more or less rapidly learn to dissociate the emotive tonus from most acts, and their maturing will proceed satisfactorily. The others will already show marked derogations from the norm, the very slight differences pointed out in infancy now being much easier to observe.

We see then that normally we try to form compulsive behavior as the rule. That is, unwittingly we try to make the child act in a certain fashion on the urge of his body tension, even though each stage of maturing necessitates the dissociation of the previously formed habit from the emotive content with which it was cultivated. This becomes a vital necessity with the onset of adolescence. The sexual function brings the young person to a state where he or she must begin to feel as an adult, and this entails an almost complete reappreciation of all the values and standards of action. The cardinal point here is the reshuffling of the affective content from the old patterns to the new ones, especially that of affection. This pattern, from the beginning, was linked with a particular person and must now become more catholic before one can feel in that spontaneous way that allows one to attach oneself to a single person more permanently. Here we meet the well-known and much-belabored subject of the mother or father complex, where the person is unable to bring about the necessary reshuffling and therefore remains to all intents and purposes impotent or frigid, never achieving full orgasm. In all such cases it turns out that the parent has established and is usually continuing to sustain the early infantile pattern of the affection being directed to one unique, irreplaceable person, such as mother or father.

The important point to make is that compulsiveness is the very thing that is methodically inculcated in the course of each person's apprenticeship, while on the other hand, the process of maturing —the loosening of the affective content from the particular objects and acts—is left to chance. We rely on "inherent intelligence," instinct, and other things that we do not know sufficiently (so that there is no danger of finding ourselves wrong for a long time to come) to help the maturing process, while we do almost everything possible to sustain the infantile dependence patterns. If the adult never matured, the whole society would be more manageable, never living its own life, but only serving the previous generation. So the new generation is raised in practice to serve the old one, children are often born to reduce the insecurity of parents, and in such cases the parents do all in their power to maintain the infantile affective patterns. The children are allowed to mature, only indirectly, because they must become economically proficient to alleviate parental insecurity. And it is this very process of becoming economically independent that gives the new generation a chance of growing up.

The process of maturing is a very subtle one, for the simple reason that we are both the molding material and steadily becoming our own molders. Nevertheless, it is worth the trouble to follow the intricacies of the process, as it gives one a clearer insight into behavior in general and enables us to assess more expediently the different methods used to readjust behavior.

From the analysis of the process of growth of a person, it may be concluded that most traditional practices are fundamentally wrong, and that entirely new methods of education must be adopted. Some people are so engrossed in the ill effects of present practices that any true perspective on the whole situation is distorted. The major problem is the lack of any clearly formulated and explicitly stated aim of education. Firstly, education, whether bad or good, channels growth and directs it into preferred grooves. Secondly, that direction uses two major means: one maintains the preferred patterns as persistently as possible, and the other excludes the rejected pattern as utterly as possible. "Thou shalt love thy father and thy mother" is as good an example as any. This precept is driven into the child with all the definiteness and thoroughness that we can imagine. All patterns undermining the precept of the sacredness of parenthood are excluded and reprimanded. Everybody is agreed that some sort of respect toward parents is necessary for the good of the children themselves, and, provided no undue harshness or excess is used, the child-parent pattern is unavoidable. Even if we decided to the contrary, the helplessness of human children in the first years of their lives would always sustain some sort of dependence relationship between children and adults, whether those adults were parents or state officials.

Now, a respectful and friendly attitude toward parents is expedient during the dependence period. However, in the adult state, when the child has reached full independence, material, emotional, physical, and intellectual, that expediency ceases to be. We can distinguish three stages in the maturing process. The first is when the pattern is so established that the child acts on it whether he wants to or not; that is, internal compulsion is established which excludes all other alternatives. The second stage is when the environmental conditions of dependence are lifted, and the expediency of compulsion is no more. The compulsive adherence to the established pattern may continue by habit if the conditioning of its establishment has been in accordance with laws governing conditioning. The pattern may be completely rejected or even reversed, love replaced by hatred, and respect by disrespect, if the compulsive pattern has been mishandled. The third stage is when maturity has been reached; that is, when the ability of dissociating emotional content or affect from any pattern has been learned. At this stage one can continue loving and respecting one's parents without internal compulsion, or equally, can continue despising and hating them without internal compulsion. In both cases the intensity of the emotive content is controllable by the person and is more dictated by the conditions than by emotional compulsiveness. Having reached that state of the ability to control dissociation of affect from action, one can see not only intellectually but also emotionally that parental love and respect are a necessity—not a law of nature, but a by-product of human experience. Behavior then becomes spontaneous and the compulsiveness is gone through the liberation of the emotional content from a unique object enforced on one in a state of physical and emotional dependence. Intellectually therefore, we understand the state of maturity as the recognition of necessity, and the freedom from the internal compulsion that accompanies the process.

The three stages from utter dependence to maturity can be clearly distinguished in all emotions, and therefore in all action, even in the learning process itself. Thus, we begin by learning because we cannot help it, we continue learning by habit or refuse to continue by rebellion, and then we learn without internal compulsion but by choice. We are helpless to begin with, and need affection; then we need it compulsively, we may continue to need it by habit or reject it by rebellion; then we free ourselves from the compulsive need for affection, and seek it through deliberate choice from the object on which we focus. We are insecure through our long dependence period; our sensation of insecurity may continue as an internal compulsion or be compulsively inverted until we are capable of dissociating the emotive content from action, and our security stops depending on our internal state and is then dependent on external circumstances.

From this point of view we can see that nothing is good or bad in itself, no pattern is harmful or perfect; it simply depends on whether the pattern reinstates itself through internal compulsion or whether we enact it in a state in which we can dissociate the emotive content from the original object to which it was linked, not through choice, but as a necessary result of our dependence. Spontaneous, mature behavior becomes possible if the learning process has taken its full course and the person has become able to direct his affective drives toward objects of his choice. He then assumes entire responsibility for his actions, and no result can compromise his ability to learn; that is, his ability to modify his attitude to the environment and, if necessary, to change his responses so that more congenial conditions obtain.

If we examine some of the most laudable things, such as perfection, progress, concentration, perseverence, regularity, methodicalness, generosity, love, or truth—we can see that in themselves they may bring complete misery to the person who enacts them through internal compulsion and to whom the alternative course is barred through fixity of the emotive content to the original object. Thus, you may find people who are incapable of seeing the futility of perfection in itself. Some will go on all their life perfecting their muscles, their memory, or whatever it may be until life is no more, without noticing that perfection is only one of the minor attributes of life. How many perfect human beings are there? How many perfect books or pictures are there? Is the rest of the world less justified in existing? Are the imperfect things not as essential to life as the perfect ones? Perfection is as essential as its opposite, and there is no justification for becoming crazy about it. As far as potent, healthy behavior goes, nothing is more important than the degree of internal compulsion with which we act. The important things will take care of themselves; we always have to eat, think and learn, have children, and die—no matter what we may believe. The *way* we do these things is the cardinal point of healthy or unsatisfactory behavior.

The shortcomings of many educators and methods are largely due to neglecting to recognize the process of maturing in its entirety. Often, therefore, remedial action is directed to the act, or to the object of the act, and not to the way it is performed. The maladjustment expresses itself not in the act or object of the act, but in the internal attitude that it brings about. It is proper to be clean, but when cleanliness is maintained through internal compulsion (that is, when uncleanliness is revulsive beyond control), it is necessary to further the arrested process of maturing until the person is capable of accepting both dirt and cleanliness with indifference.

In every stable set of conditions, there is a certain optimum of maturity that is desirable and is achieved by a considerable number of people. If one or another important conditions is changed, the maturing process must be set going again. Maturity is not a state reached with age or experience—it is a process that goes on until death in all evolving and creative people. Unfortunately, we often nip it in the bud. Through shortsightedness, we think that because a given pattern or attitude is good or useful to human society, if not to the person himself, we can fix it into his behavior with a definiteness that will make him a sure victim of any considerable deviation from the norm of his personal experience. The rigor with which we inculcate the rigidness of Human Nature is the main source of our misery. The human nervous system is the least rigid of all structures; it grows and forms itself while we undergo experience. It is more affected by personal experience than the nervous system of any other animal. Personal experience is the key to our "greatness" and to our misery.

The aim of readjustment emerges very clearly from our discussion. It is not making a person conscious of the reasons and events that led him to adopt a given attitude or pattern of action, although such realizations may help him to restart the maturing process from its point of arrested immobility. It is not making a person aware of the defects in our social traditions and customs, which are often quite irrational and need sweeping away at the earliest opportunity, which is always right now. This may help him to readjust himself into another stable configuration, but it will still leave him a limping cripple with a nice prothesis instead of a simple crutch. And it is not to give him an insight into the inner workings of his behavior, although this too is a great help. For there are millions who are completely unaware of their early experiences, who are convinced that everything in society is simply divinely perfect, who have no insight into the inner processes of their behavior, and yet they are capable of steering their ship through the storm without faltering and without ever needing the emotional support of another person. The mature adult, who is capable of taking responsibility for his own life, has one thing that he has learned, and that is how to dissociate emotion from patterns established under the stress of dependence and to fix the urge for action on what he finds expedient. Because of the control achieved in shifting the emotive content, its intensity is equally under his control. This is implicitly contained in the previously mentioned aims of education and is often acted upon unwittingly —hence their erratic successes. The clear perception of the goal makes aiming something that can be learned, and *mis* aiming obvious.

In short, all functioning involving the human cortex follows lines similar to those concerned with language. At birth no connections exist that can be activated by volition (controlled by the individual) to produce speech. The baby can only activate his vocal cords in a reflective fashion, and there is great similarity among the cries of different babies. The individual differences are not greater than those of other reflexes. Personal experience forms certain connections, and these are compulsive in character whether the adult is kind or not. Their compulsiveness is a result of the dependence relationship of a helpless baby and an adult, in which the action, or its inhibition, obtained by an increased flow of affection and friendliness is still compulsive in the sense that it is not spontaneous. Gradually all the unwanted sounds are weeded out, and the desired ones are fostered to confrom to the language of the adults.

In the beginning, therefore, every utterance is linked with a certain affect. Later some dissociation of the original affects from the patterns learned takes place, and the adolescent becomes capable of personal expressions, although on the whole there is little adolescent departure from parental patterns. Maturity of this function is achieved when a person learns to dissociate completely thought from particular words, as well as the affect linked with them, and transfer to a new set of words forming a complete new language. The three steps from dependence to maturity for any function can clearly be seen in the verbal function, if thought is compared with the emotive urge for action, and the actual performance to the words used.

The part played by personal experience in action is particularly noticeable here. People who have not learned a foreign language feel that their personality was intended for their mother tongue only. All children, however, who were not constrained to one language only speak two or three languages in early childhood. In the same manner, it is possible to dissociate the original affect from any pattern of doing and form new ones well into middle age.

If we examine any concrete case of functional impotence—that is, inability to act without any detectable anatomical reason and in spite of strong desire to perform—we find that the main complaint is invariably accompanied by one or another of the following: digestive disorders, improper breathing, offensive smells from the mouth, the nose, and fecal matter, faulty posture, unbalanced muscular control, vertigo and dizziness in rotation and swinging, vascular disorders such as abnormal blushing and perspiring, poor friendship relations, matrimonial difficulties, impaired vision, and feet trouble. All these disorders are present in some degree, and some are more or less pronounced in one or the other person. We can understand, therefore, why and how *all* methods bring about relief in *some* cases, and often produce considerable improvement. There is no disease here, in the usual sense of the word, but an improperly constructed personality with improper controls. Some domains or planes of activity may even be exceptionally well developed; indeed, that is the positive and useful counterpart to the general lack of balance and cohesion of the entire personality structure. Moreover, this counterdevelopment is the clue to the contradictory and conflicting sets of habits of thought, drives, and actions. The person bends all his vitality into the planes of activity in which he is capable of potent action; that is, in the planes in which maturation is least impeded.

IMPROVING ACTION

To improve action, we must find at each stage what is the detail that will bring about the greatest improvement. In body acts it is generally very difficult to find these details, because the mental state and the body attitude and function feel like one thing, and not at all as made up of parts that can be influenced or altered individually.

After a number of repeated performances, the whole act and the sensations accompanying it become one inseparable unit, which cannot be subdivided into elementary constituents. Even the sensation of effort we feel, and the resistance to starting or continuing, become part of the act and essential to its accomplishment. One becomes readily aware of this component when examining any physical act that we can perform moderately well. Try sawing, for instance, or using a file—you will feel quite distinctly that you are producing not only the action that you intend to produce, but also that part of the action that hinders the intended action and causes the feeling of resistance and effort.

If you carefully observe a person who is an expert in this particular action, however, you will find that he seems to do much less than when you try your hand at it. He does in fact omit all the acts that are not necessary for moving the saw or the file. At the same time, he does not seem to feel that he makes an effort, and also seems to meet no resistance. Another important thing can be observed, though not so easily: he does make little special actions with the hands and arms, but initiates the forward and backward motions with his hips. The arms move mostly together with the body and change direction with it, and the relative motion of the arms to the body is only secondary.

It is very important to realize that incompetence does not mean lack of the essential action for achieving the end, but consists largely in enacting unnecessary, parasitic acts. Unaware, we enact all that is sensed as resistance. The incompetent man produces so much unnecessary and often contradictory action that the intended act is accompanied with an overwhelming sense of resistance. Sometimes this resistance seems so great that the tension requiring release must be very great indeed to force the person to further attempts.

Thus, some people invariably complicate the sexual act with economic, moral, and other considerations that turn it into a task accompanied by intense extraneous feelings. Nobody can dwell on these ideas without uneasiness, for they contain fundamental contradictions—especially if one has had an unbalanced religious upbringing. The feeling of conflict is carried on to the main sexual act and becomes habitual. This sensation of conflict, which has nothing to do with the act itself, is sometimes so strongly linked to it as to invariably appear together with it, and to remain present until physical action is in progress. At that moment the sensation of conflict often disappears completely.

The origin of this linkage of sex with extraneous feelings lies in the fact that sexual activity is checked by society for many years after we become physiologically fit for it. And during those years, we are repeatedly made aware that only after solving the problem of dependence have we the "right" to sexual relations. During the many years of imposed continence, social, moral, economic, and religious factors mold our attitude to persons of the opposite sex, toward whom we feel sexually inclined, and thus prepare and form the linkage of the conflict with sex. Only potent people—those who have matured and learned to dissociate habitual patterns of their previous experience and to use only those parts that are necessary for the task at hand—become, after some apprenticeship, capable of satisfactory action.

To get rid of incompetence, one must learn to distinguish the parasitic elements that one enacts unaware, by habit, and thus become a real adult. The competent adult's action is so simple that he can never understand the complexity that bewilders the incompetent person, who erroneously tries to achieve (without knowing how to throw overboard the impeding ballast) an action that needs poised simplicity and serenity of attitude. The most competent adult would break down had he to labor under the same conditions.

To be of any practical use, the mode of doing must not be ideal but expedient—one that can be normally used in our present-day society. It is useless to aspire to an ideal of being better than everybody else. The main object is to form an attitude and a new set of responses that permit an even and poised application of oneself to the business of living and not to create new terrain for conflict. Moreover, the new mode of action must perforce be adjusted to the *present* environment—even though everybody agrees that our social structure and our education need radical improvement if they are to become suitable for a society of creative, evolving, mature adults.

12. Correct Posture

As already discussed, posture relates to action, and not to the maintenance of any given position. *Acture* would perhaps be a better word for it. The appropriateness of *acture* can be judged from two standpoints generally leading to opposite conclusions. If we focus our attention on the action to be achieved, most people act correctly and their body posture is the best possible, considering the means and knowledge at their disposal. A child who must sit on chairs that are not carefully designed for her age, without due apprenticeship in sitting, consequently experiences insufficient development of the muscles of the pelvic joints (because our distorted notions of hygiene eliminate crawling much too soon, with the premium of affection and praise put on early attempts at standing, etc.). She does, in fact, the best she can when she sits with her head slumping forward and her spine curved. As Bengt Akerblom has amply proved in his book *Standing and Sitting,* this sort of sitting involves little muscular tension, the weight of the body being supported by the ligaments of the spine. Considering the demands made on children when they begin to go to school —to sit still for a rather long stretch without any previous preparation for such a difficult task—any position of the body that will give them the possibility of achieving what is required from them must be (and, in fact, is) considered as correct action.

On the other hand if we focus attention on the posture or *acture* (the way an action is accomplished and the way it can best be accomplished by a human being) most people make absurdly bad use of themselves.

It is alleged by teachers and physical culturists that bad posture is harmful. I venture to brave this opinion as ill-conceived. There is no general harm whatsoever in any awkward or ungainly configuration of the body in itself, except the minor local effect. A well-coordinated person can adopt any position for any length of time without the ill effects that accompany the same configuration in those who do so (as they would put it) naturally. The ill effect that we do find is not due to an anatomical configuration that is harmful per se, but to the fact that it is compulsive and is the only one the ill-coordinated person uses for performing the act. Thus an asthmatic holds her chest, throat, and head in a special configuration to which she reverts continuously. From all the possible alignments of these body segments, she is constrained to use only one, which the well-coordinated person can adopt at will with only very minor inconveniences and without becoming an asthmatic at that. This exclusion of alternative use is obviously compulsive. The pattern of doing that has brought the person to this state is the harm-producing agent, not the anatomical configuration. And, in fact, as soon as the compulsiveness is lifted there is no asthmatic state any more.

The bad posture of the asthmatic is the best choice possible in the continuous fear of abandonment in which she lives, as long as she has not learned to be emotionally self-sufficient. She has been submitted to a persistent scotch shower of intense affection and alienation at a time when she could not possibly face abandonment without the overwhelming sense of anxiety that reflectively shrinks the body. In the body's quest for safety, the flexor muscles are tensed and the extensors inhibited. This is the reaction to falling in all onsets of fear. The lowering of the head and the sinking of the chest are the best movements to protect the body from the injury expected to come from above, when flight is unthinkable and hitting back utterly inhibited (as it would be for a small child facing her parents). And so long as this attitude of fear of abandonment is sustained by personal experience of the individual, that posture remains the best possible. She will revert to it in any sudden onslaught of circumstances demanding a fighting response to a powerful opponent; that is, in all circumstances in which she feels abandoned and left alone to fight her battles.

Thus, it is the emotional immaturity that is the harmful agent, not the particular posture, as this emotional attitude reinstates compulsively the situation for which the asthmatic response and the asthmatic posture are a necessity. The strong emotional forces involved during the dependence period have prevented the person from attaining varied, spontaneous self-use and from exploring the full range of her abilities. These forces have perpetuated an attitude and configuration that proved to be effective in that period to the exclusion of any other.

Correct posture has little useful meaning without consideration of the state of maturity, the situation, the emotional means, and the state of the body. It is generally very far from what it could be if compulsiveness were eliminated. Remember that compulsiveness, as it is used here, refers to the way in which the habit of behavior has been formed under the duress of affection, security, and the allied emotional agents, that are to the child the means of earning her livelihood. This does not necessarily mean severe punishment and harshness (which are, however, not excluded) either.

In the properly matured individual, activity is spontaneous in all familiar circumstances and potent when a more refined control is required. The spontaneity and the potency are possible because the mature adult has learned to dissociate emotions from body patterns, she has lifted compulsiveness from her behavior, and she makes her habits in accordance with what she deems necessary or desirable. This lifting of compulsiveness from behavior results in greater freedom and independence, similar to the recognition of necessity that lifts the compulsiveness from social behavior.

Correct posture is a matter of emotional growth and learning. It is not acquired by simple exercising or by repetition of the desired act or attitude. Learning is not a purely mental occupation, as many people believe, just as the acquisition of skill is not a purely physical process. Essentially, it consists in recognizing in the total situation—environment, mind, and body—a relationship in the form of a sensation that in the long run becomes so distinct that we can almost describe it in sensible language. The earliest learning consists in the exploration of our own body possibilities to move and act. In the multitude of undifferentiated muscular contractions, we soon learn to recognize configurations that have a bearing, a meaning, or relatedness to the exterior world of which our body is a part. Slowly these recognitions become definite acts. In this way, we learn to walk, to speak, and to use a spoon. To acquire better posture, it is necessary to restart and further this process of learning, and bring it to a higher level of excellence.

In any coordinated, well-learned action—such as thinking, speaking, eating, breathing, solving problems, drawing, or fighting —we can distinguish certain features or recognize the following sensations:

1. *Absence of effort.* In good action, the sensation of effort is absent no matter what the actual expenditure of energy is. Much of our action is so poor that this assertion sounds utterly preposterous. It suffices, however, to observe a good judo man, an expert weight lifter, a figure-skating champion, a first-class acrobat, a great diva, an Arabian horseman, a skillful porter—in fact, anybody who has learned to perform correctly mental or bodily actions—in order to convince oneself that the sensation of effort is the subjective feeling of wasted movement. All inefficient action is accompanied by this sensation; it is a sign of incompetence. When carefully analyzed, it is always possible to show convincingly that the sensation of effort is due to other actions being enacted besides the one intended.

Externally, the sensation of effort can be identified through hardly perceptible breaks in the breathing rhythm, poor performances, halting of breath, kinks in the curvature of the spine (that develop from uneven bending or twisting of the vertebrae, where some are being held rigidly in groups with only one or two bending or twisting to the possible limit of ligament stretch), and unnecessary fixation of joints in space (too abrupt transference of motion from one joint to another). We shall see later the means of reducing these and innumerable other details to a single attitude.

2. *The absence of resistance.* When there is external objective resistance (such as that presented by the corner of a cathedral to motion) no displacement takes place and no work is done. The sensation of effort is the greatest possible, with efficiency being zero.

The sensation of resistance is produced by conflicting impulses arriving at the voluntary skeletal muscles. The voluntary control is dictating one state and configuration of muscular contraction for the projected act, while the balance of the body is being maintained in a configuration incompatible with the act to be achieved. In all such cases, the body is actively prevented from adjusting itself to the better alignment by a voluntary act of standing or sitting that is so habitual that the person reverts to it without ever doubting its adequacy.

Resistance is sensed together with muscular tension even when the act involves such a little change in body space as does simply thinking. Normally we try to remedy the situation by a further effort of "will." Whenever will effort is necessary, there is unrecognized cross motiviation, and this is an extremely wasteful method of obtaining results. Only immature people need will effort to act. The mature person clears up all the irrelevant motivations and uses interest, necessity, and skill unhindered by unrecognized emotional urges. This ability of inhibiting the distracting tendencies is acquired by the mature person through careful and painstaking learning of her own functioning. (Stiffening of the jaws for instance—which enacts doubt of ability to do—does not invent, create, or do anything, it only accompanies a sufficient expense of energy to arrive at an end in spite of the bad coordination of motivation and muscle.)

The sensation of resistance is due to an improper inhibition and integration of the urges to action before enacting them. It is essentially a sign of infantile manipulation of motivation. The keener the watch on resistance, the finer is the skill and competence in the end. This rule holds good for thinking, sex, feeling, and acting in general. Needless to say, this watching is only necessary during the learning period. Later the self-image in action already contains all the details of proper attitude and posture as part of an undivided whole. Revision and conscious intervention are necessary in entirely new situations only.

The sensation of resistance coincides with a particular fault in the distribution of contraction in the musculature. The power-producing muscles are located around the pelvis. The muscles of the limbs only place the bones in such a relationship as to transmit the power moving the body. They direct the transmission of power most of the time, but are not the major source of it. In correct *acture,* no matter what the movement is—standing up, sitting down, pushing or pulling—power is transmitted from the pelvic joints through the spine to the head. The contractions along the spine are only synergetic (just enough to hold the spine in the position adequate for power transmission), and there is no voluntary contraction of the muscles of the head-neck joints unless this is the object of the action. The sensation of resistance arises when the limbs, the chest, the shoulders, or another part of the body is made to do the job of the pelvic and abdominal muscles.

The question of resistance is of utmost importance: firstly, because in ignoring it we continue acting against ourselves while believing ourselves to be conquering objective difficulties; secondly, because without a conscious awareness of resistance we can never get rid of it before we meet with major catastrophes or risks; thirdly, because when we see other people succeeding where we fail even though we try our best, we ascribe to ourselves in self-protection some unfortunate inborn defect and turn away from the activity. Repeated admissions of this sort sap vitality; they are the product of a tired and tried imagination and have little to do with objective reality.

3. *The presence of reversibility.* The main feature of correct *acture* or posture in all procedures depending on and existing within the scope of voluntary action is reversibility. At every instant or stage of a correct act, it can be stopped, withheld from continuing, or reversed without any preliminary change of attitude and without effort. The qualifications of this rule take into account reflex action and inertia as in swallowing or jumping. When the swallowing reflex is started, the propulsion of food is no longer within the scope of voluntary control. When we leave the ground with both feet, we lose control to a large extent. It may be interesting to note that control of swallowing and regurgitation can be acquired, and expert yogis can do so at will. Also, expert jumpers continue

having a considerable measure of control over their flight through the air, thanks to rapid change in the moment of inertia of the body, produced by comparatively small changes in the body's configuration.

In a temper, in a state of anxiety, hilarity, shame, or guilt—in short, in all cases of emotional tension of high tone where our action is compulsive—reversibility is compromised so completely that the question of correctness no longer has any meaning.

Reversibility is a feature of all correct action, even sleep. Thus, the well-coordinated mature person, such as found among people who have succeeded in making their occupation their pleasure, can go off to sleep when he feels like it and wake up when necessary. Moreover, all healthy animals and humans do not object to being awakened, as they can stop sleeping and resume sleeping without trouble. The ability to stop an action, a process, restart it, reverse it, or drop it altogether is one of the finer criteria of proper *acture.* Only really mature and well-coordinated people can interrupt intercourse, give it up, or resume it without any trouble. The importance of reversibility is that it is possible only when there is fine control of excitation and inhibition and a normal ebb and flow between the parasympathetic and the sympathetic. The test of reversibility holds good for all human activity whether it is viewed from the physical or the emotional standpoint.

4. *Breathing and incorrect posture.* Holding the breath is the clearest observable sign of incorrect posture or *acture.* Many people hold their breath in one way or another. The body image they have formed is such that they have to produce a preparatory rearrangement of their throat, chest, and abdomen before they can speak or initiate any motion whatsoever. In some the disturbance is so manifest that the chest is fixed in the position of inspiration or expiration continuously. The normal ventilation is upset, with profound effects on the acid-base balance of the blood.

In conditions of extreme alkalinity of the blood, the muscles contract indiscriminately at the slightest stimulus coming from the outside, or at the initiation of any act, and tetanization takes place. In extreme acidity, as in diabetes, no muscular response can be elicited; there is a state of coma. The alkalinity of the blood can be markedly increased by excessive loss of carbon dioxide; exhaling forcibly by blowing for about two minutes brings about an increased neuromuscular excitability, which is first detectable in the region of the mouth and fingers.

The phenomenon is complex. For example, if the exhaling is done, not by blowing, but by sharp pushes forward of the lower abdominal muscles (as a dog does when barking), no inconvenience is observed even after prolonged repetition. Habitual faulty holding of the breath is normally found together with muscular excitability, and vice versa. Reciprocity seems to be necessary for any function that is a continuous process.

At first sight, the four features of correct posture seem to contradict common experience and to confirm it only occasionally. Some simple, ever recurring, ordinary movements are in fact performed practically before we are aware of doing anything at all. On the other hand, most action that needs any conscious decision before we engage it generally produces all the faulty sensations and states that we have just enumerated. Sometimes we find ourselves in a special state that generally coincides with ease of mind and happiness; during such fleeting moments, posture is in much better agreement with our requirements. To understand this and to give us a clearer picture of the functioning of the human frame, it is necessary to know something of the special features of the human skeleton and the functioning of the musculature.

If we look at the human skeleton, we notice that the trunk and head are connected to the pelvis by the rather slender pillar of the lumbar spine. At the junction with the pelvis, we find the largest vertebrae, on which are piled vertebrae that gradually decrease in size up to the last two—the atlas and the axis—on which the head is articulated. If we remember that muscles can only create tension and therefore produce mostly pulling actions, the spine resembles a mainstay that is held in position by muscles anchored at the pelvis as its base. The resultant pull at any instant must pass through the base of the column, and its direction must be continuous along the main direction of the spine. The direction of the resultant pull can deviate from the direction of the spine only slightly if the strain that tends to make the vertebrae slide on one another and stretch the ligaments to the point of damage is to be prevented.

The thoracic cage, the shoulders, and the arms are suspended from the spine. In order to open the cage or lift the arms, muscles having one end inserted higher than the other must come into action. It is important to realize this, as well as to realize that all other muscles fixed to the ribs with one end higher and the other one lower cannot but have a fixing effect on the cage that generally pulls it downward and reduces the volume inside of it.

The head rides on top of the column. Its center of gravity is in front of the point of support and falls forward and down, until the chin rests on the chest bone if the muscles of the neck are severed. It is not necessary to know anything at all about muscles and skeleton to use them properly, but it saves time and is very useful to have a working idea of the body in order to learn an improved use of it.

In quadrupeds, such as horses, cattle, or deer, the head is very heavy and hangs at the end of a horizontally protruding neck. The muscles holding this awkward and heavy structure behave differently from what we know through experience about muscular work. These animals hold their heads in a horizontal (or rest) position for extremely long periods without the slightest sign of fatigue. From this rest position, of the head, we can see the animal lifting it higher when a suspicious noise reaches it or lowering it to eat and drink. The lowered position of the head needs less contraction of the muscles of the neck. Yet this is more tiring to the animal, which lifts its head every now and then to the normal position for a rest. This is odd when one begins to think about it, yet we usually find it quite sensible, for we do very similar things. Our head too, has its center of gravity in front of its support, yet our neck never becomes tired enough so that the head drops forward from muscular fatigue. Also the center of gravity of the whole body when projected onto the ground falls in front of the ankle joint at least half an inch and up to about two inches. Yet the calf muscles that hold the tibias and prevent the body from going down and forward around the ankle joint never feel the effort at all. We feel tiredness elsewhere long before the calf muscles are fatigued. However, we can fatigue the calf muscles quite easily and in a very short time by making them work otherwise than to support the body in the standing position. The same holds true for our neck muscles.

We see, therefore, that there are two kinds of muscular contractions. One kind is involved in intense, slow, sustained effort; the other is of graded intensity—faster, but of much shorter duration. Of the first kind, we have no awareness at all. The second is entirely obedient to our volition and produces inner awareness. The first is tonic contraction, and the second is the phasic contraction which we use through direct voluntary control in all our acts.

The tone in tonically contracted muscles is produced primarily by the weight of the segments pulling on the muscles, which prevents the segments from yielding to gravitational pull. This pull causes the nerve fibers embedded in the muscles to send out impulses that travel toward some lower centers and result in the contraction of the muscles on arrival. All this traffic of impulses interests the lower parts of the nervous system, and does not affect the higher cortical centers except very indirectly. The tonic distribution of the contraction of the skeletal muscles is an evolutionary adaptation of the human organism to the gravitational field of the earth and is only indirectly influenced by each individual personal experience.

The impulses initiating the voluntary contractions of the skeletal muscles originate in the cortex and reach the spinal cord by passing the pyramidal tract, which is a connecting bundle of fibers. The spinal cord then sends the impulses that actually contract the muscles. Before the pyramidal tract has grown down into the spine, no voluntary action is possible in the segments below.

Each skeletal muscle has two sorts of fibers, red ones and pale ones. The red fibers contract slowly and fatigue even more slowly; the pale ones contract sharply and fatigue rapidly. Voluntary movements correspond, therefore, to the pale fibers' contractions, and tonic movements to the red ones. Muscles that are constantly tonically contracted and do the major work of maintaining the body against gravitational pull—that is, all the muscles extending the articulations, the *extensors,* which are also referred to as "anti-gravity muscles"—have more red fibers than the *flexor* muscles, which contract much faster.

The voluntary movements are due to impulses from the highest nervous centers, which have an overriding control over the lower centers. Thus the horse can inhibit the tonic contraction of its neck extensors and voluntarily lower its head or enhance them and lift its head. When the voluntary impulses stop arriving, the head returns to its normal position, as the inhibitory effect on the tonic contraction is lifted. That is, when the horse does nothing at all its head is lifted by the tonic apparatus that evolved with its species adaptation to the physical environment.

In human beings, the voluntary movements are essentially the result of personal experience, as in speaking, where the connection patterns or paths of the different cortical cells are most obviously formed in correspondence with the immediate environment, unlike the tonic apparatus, which is the result of adaptation of the species. The increased flexor activity, which can only flex articulations and generally shorten the stature, has therefore something to do with the personal experience of the individual. It is useful to keep in mind that flexors and extensors are, as the physiologist puts it, *agonists* and *antagonists.* That is, they cooperate in a seesaw manner: when the flexors shorten a limb, the extensors yield and lengthen to allow voluntary action to take place, and at the same time create the rigidity required of the limb. It is also important to note that the fibers of the autonomic (or vegetative, or the sympathetic and parasympathetic) nervous system innervate most of the muscles so that the viscera affect and are affected by the general body configuration.

We have now reached a point of capital importance in the understanding of *acture* or posture. Namely, if in the act of standing we eliminate all contraction due to impulses from the cortical areas (such as are subject to volition in the physiological sense—that is, with no concern as to whether we are aware of issuing the order producing the contraction or whether its origin is entirely unknown to us) the body will be held in the tonically erect posture that the evolutionary adaptation of the skeleton, muscles, and the tonic apparatus of the nervous system has produced.

This unexpected conclusion can be substantiated by making any person aware of his or her body in space, of habitual contractions that have become second nature, of skeletal configuration, and in general by reeducating the kinesthetic sense. With each appreciation and correction of the voluntarily controllable muscles and joints, and with the ensuing ability not to do the particular acts of which in the past we were unaware, the body increases in length, the stature becomes more erect, and the joints, spine, and head tend toward the ideal configuration. The body feels lighter and lighter until one feels as if one were walking on air.

The ideal standing posture is obtained not by doing something to oneself, but by literally doing nothing, that is, by eliminating all acts of voluntary origin due to motivations other than standing that have become automatic and are now part and parcel of the personal *acture* of the situation of standing.

The ideal configuration cannot be reached immediately. The management of voluntary *acture* can be improved faster than can the management of the *acture* of the joints and vertebrae, the hipjoints, the toes and others in which movement has been eliminated for a long period of time. Such joints have formed spongy fibrous textures that were necessary to help to maintain the habitual configuration without overtaxing the voluntary muscular mechanisms, which are ill-suited for such monotonous and unchanging holding of position. The deformations disappear relatively rapidly as soon as they are no longer sustained continuously.

We have seen that the lumbar spine is the only bony and rigid link between the pelvis and the trunk and also that longitudinal stresses are those that are best transmitted through the spine when no other muscular activity is present except tonic contractions. The spine then assumes a smoothly wavering line, and each vertebra is in full contact with both the one below it and the one above it. In movements bending and twisting the spine, it is essential that the bend or twist should interest as many vertebrae as necessary so that no vertebra undergoes exceptional stresses approaching the limit of movement safeguarded by the ligaments. The permanent immobilization of some groups of vertebrae shifts the strain onto the remaining ones, which then work nearer to the limit of safety (with numerous ill effects, both mechanical and to the general health).

All voluntary direction for using oneself contracts the muscles, and one of two possibilities can result. First, the final result of the contraction at every instant is such that the main forces through the spine (the only force transmitting solid connection between the trunk and the pelvis) remain essentially longitudinal and continue all along it in the direction of the spine. If this remains true at every instant and at every point of the spine, we obtain the best possible *acture* from every point of view: efficiency, grace, ease, and coordination. Such *acture* makes learning of skills an easy and self-maintaining process.

The second possibility is that the instantaneous total result of the muscular contraction is not transmitted efficiently along the spine, but is made up of forces that tend to shear or fold it. Only one component of such force is then transmitted through the solid lumbar link, with the ligaments preventing the actual shear or bent from taking place. To enable the body to comply with the voluntary direction, we contract ourselves not only for the purpose of the voluntary act but also to maintain the habitually peculiar bents and twists of the spine while performing the act. The *acture* is inefficient, because of the dash-dot effect that the different joints have when the vertebrae are gaping or when the curve of the spine is pronounced. The configuration is ungainly, the movement heavy and uncoordinated, as the trunk does not move as one whole in the direction of the intended motion—but only parts of it—while others actually move in the opposite direction.

Before passing on to illustrate the preceding with particular acts, I would like to insist on a point that has already been made:

namely, improper *acture* is so widespread and occurs so much more frequently than the proper one, that it is impossible to agree with the generally held opinion of some inherent weakness or carelessness or degeneration in such persons. My experience as a judo teacher extended over twenty-five years and has included nearly 5,000 people of different races and nationalities, mostly young and strong men and women, each individual being under my observation for years on end. This experience has convinced me that there is little foundation for such opinions, except in a very small number of clearly pathological cases. In all the others, the bad use is the result of great vitality and adjustability to demands that society in its ignorance makes on its growing members without paying any attention to the means at the command of the individual, let alone the need to provide proper ones.

All incorrect *acture* can be traced back to premature or too violent demands made on the person. The contractions that are maintained in all action as a personal manner of doing, irrespective of the act, always express an emotional attitude. The attitude found most frequently is that of insecurity or the masquerade of ignoring it. Physiologically stiffening the body, lowering the head, sinking the chest, contracting and flattening the abdomen—when performed not in the course of a purposeful action, but as acts in themselves—are protective acts. The reactions to falling (protection of the head from overhead threats; protection of the throat, the pit of the stomach, the soft "underbelly," the genitals) are all produced by flexor contraction and are all effective measures that give a sense of relative security in face of sudden or great danger. They either offer a hard, bony obstacle to the threat, or they withdraw the vulnerable soft organ as far as possible. The flexor contraction is inhibitory to extensors, and insufficient tone in the antigravity extensors is the resultant rule in bad posture.

Bad *acture* may be due to doubt, fear, hesitation, guilt, shame, or impotence. Or to other emotional attitudes formed in one's personal experience of the world, all depending on the kind of security the environment has brought the individual to consider as essential for her safety. For some, the crucial factor will be lack of affection, for some lack of approval, lack of personal beauty, lack of aggressiveness, lack of physical strength—lack of something or other that the person has learned to consider as essential for her as a human being.

The actual *acture* is complicated by the fact that most people become aware of a difference between their own *acture* and that of their idols in early youth or adolescence. It is generally then that the compensatory, masquerading business takes place. The adolescents notice the outstanding differences and try to remedy them by an appropriate direction of themselves. As we have seen, no voluntary direction can correct bad posture; however, it does change the appearance of the body—not by lifting the contraction that needs lifting, but by enacting a compensatory one. The segment changes its appearance and *looks* roughly as it should, but not without the strain of voluntary action. By constant vigilance and self-reminding, one learns to maintain two conflicting contractions. The results are exclusion of movement in the parts under conscious focusing, rigidity and muscular tenseness, halting of breath, and all the rest of it. In the long run the pattern becomes habitual, semiautomatic, and familiar to the point of being considered as one's own nature, but only at the expense of strain and nervous exhaustion. The body pattern formed under emotional stress is maintained without any further question of its validity, and the emotional attitude is reinstated and sustained by the body pattern as part of the whole situation, so that emotional maturity on that plane is hindered. The person feels bewitched, for she often makes frantic efforts to shake herself out of the lethargic stagnation into which her emotional development has been arrested, only to find herself back where she was because of the vicious reciprocity which the total situation has created between the body patterns and the emotions in the higher centers.

When a young girl is told to be ashamed of herself because of her growing breasts becoming conspicuous, especially if it is her mother who tells her this, she does feel ashamed and tries her best to make them inconspicuous. She holds her chest at the extreme position of breathing out and keeps it motionless, excluding all movement of the clavicles and the sternum. Her neck becomes longer and longer, voice more highly pitched, breasts flabby and hanging, arms toneless, breathing shallow and metabolism low, with fat gathering in the part of the body from which mobility is excluded and so forth. In short, her *acture* is compulsive, because she has lost the ability of voluntary control over some parts of herself and limited the range of numerous articulations to one compulsively exclusive pattern. She feels guilty by her own admission but through no fault of her own; the world seems hostile to her, as it punishes her cruelly. But a mother's observations of that sort can produce such effects only on a girl in whom an excessive need for affection and approval has been carefully fostered earlier. Such a person has inhibited spontaneity and has a compulsive need to be good. The amount of suffering she knows nobody really can fathom. The inadequacy of physical training by itself is quite obvious. She must also learn that conspicuous breasts need not and cannot be removed, and that anything she can do to hide them will only make them only more conspicuous to everybody whom it may concern.

Similar postural disturbances are produced by having small breasts, and by any other part of the body, because there is no norm for perfection. Pushing the analysis further, we find that postural maladjustment is in fact the result of adjustment to society dictated by an overdeveloped emotional urge, that distorts objective appreciation of real values. At the bottom of maladjustment is essential ignorance. And I can clearly see unmistakable signs of general improvement. *Already the new generation is incomparably better handled, and the future will be even brighter, atom bomb or no atom bomb. When compulsive behavior is eliminated and there is a greater proportion of potency in men and women, it will be used, as has always been the case, for increasing human security, not for destroying it.*

To make any modification in behavior into a start for further development, we must first eliminate all sources of irritation that lead to heightened emotional tone, which greatly hinders self-direction in any but the most familiar ways. If the new modes of action are tried in the presence of pain or discomfort, they have little chance of being sought after with any eagerness. Instead, the pain or discomfort will reinstate the old habits and will bring to nought all learning. Corns, ingrown toenails, and other sources of discomfort must be eliminated before starting. The usual means are only temporary. They will not eliminate the trouble, because the exaggerated sensitivity of the feet, their flatness, and other troubles are not unconnected with behavior. They are sustained by the person's attitude and manner of doing. One picks tight shoes to conceal the width of the feet, to look smart, noble, or delicate. One walks in a particularly inappropriate manner for reasons dictated by a distorted dependence relationship to other people. Every problem has some extraneous motive besides the mechanical source of trouble. All the problems together form a coherent complex. They are the core of the complaint, and they will disappear together in due course. For the moment, they must be dealt with in the usual way in order to obtain temporary relief.

Similarly, constipation must be attended to from the start. Obviously there is no panacea treatment, but the following suggestions may be of considerable assistance for general improvement. People with long bodies relative to their legs may find a vegetable diet much more congenial. On the other hand, people with short bodies relative to their legs may find the elimination, or at least the reduction, of rough cellulose in their daily diet brings better results. Also, adopting the squatting position (as when using Turkish toilet rooms) instead of sitting is more congenial for defecation and often yields surprisingly good results, especially if the naked thighs are allowed to touch the naked skin of the chest and abdomen. It is also good to drink fluids after meals and as little as possible during them. Another stratagem is to separate protein intake from starch as much as possible.

The next important area that bears the marks of distorted dependence, and sustains the present symptoms, is feeding. The food intake habits must be rational. They are certainly not so in most cases. We have in mind the emotional attitude toward food and the alimentary hygiene of the individual child. Her food habits have been formed in the early stages of dependence and always serve some other purpose in addition to feeding. For example, she feels that somebody must know that she has not eaten or that she has indigestion, and she feels that somebody else must not know these things. A habitual pattern of guilt can be detected when we pay attention to the frequency of digestive malaise that the child knows to be due to what she has eaten or eaten too much of. The fact that she knows what the cause of her discomfort is shows that she cannot stop herself from doing what she knows to be wrong; she is acting under a compulsion. Her efforts fail because the compulsion is unrecognized and therefore cannot be affected by what she does. What she does is thus punishing, because she feels guilty and deserving of suffering. We shall see later when dealing with cross motivation in general how to solve this problem.

Another important point that needs immediate attention is the offensive smell from the mucous openings of the body—the mouth, the nose, the throat, the ears, the anus, and (in women) the vagina. These smells are often responsible for loneliness and marital indifference, for the simple reason that nobody has the courage to point them out to the offender. It is necessary to make certain, by objective testing, whether one smells offensively. The best approach is to ask whether one is an offender or not. During menstruation and during periods of depression, the odor of most excretions of all people becomes more offensive than usual. One should take notice of the increased smell of the stool and urine to check all the others. During attack periods, more frequent washing than normal hygiene requires is absolutely necessary, and, of course, medical advice should be sought without delay.

Perhaps posture is the most important field where a change is required in all cases of distorted dependence. There is certainly unnecessary tension in the pelvis muscles and the neck, as well as flabbiness in the antagonists of the contracted muscles. I consider posture so important that much of this book is concerned with it.

But considerable as these changes may be, it is also indispensable to support them by teaching better control and coordination, so that the learner does not have to fall back on habitual poor control for want of an alternative. All these means are intended to help to make the reinstatement of anxiety rare to begin with and impossible in the end. Nothing furthers the formation of the correct attitude more than the dissipation of anxiety. Maladjustment is not a disease, but the result of wrong learning or the learning of wrong methods. Realizing this fact alone should lift sufficient weight off the shoulders that carry it.

Perhaps it is worthwhile to say explicitly what is understood by this alternative resting on one foot and then on the other—constipation and compulsion—physical ailment on one hand and emotional trouble on the other. Most people agree that chronic constipation may have its accompanying irritability and moods, but they generally decide that going to the doctor, or the nature cure practitioner, or the osteopath, or whoever it may be who will reduce the trouble is good enough. They feel that once the irksome symptom has disappeared they have cleared up the trouble. Everybody knows that stomach ulcers have some connection with worry, but in spite of the psychosomatic component the treatment still usually consists of a diet and potential surgical intervention, *or* of psychological treatment. The treatment is generally *either* one *or* the other for the simple reason that there really are no psychosomatic methods of treatment yet.

13. The Means at Our Disposal

There is a lot of truth in the saying that we understand ourselves worse than anybody else. The more we see a thing the more obvious it becomes to us, whether we know it or not. When faced with the problem of readjusting ourselves, we are at once at a loss for a starting point. No sooner have we decided on one thing when we see a more important one. It is difficult to know precisely the spot where clarity is most needed.

First we must understand very clearly the relationship of emotions, mental thinking, and body action. By *emotion* we mean not only the exacerbation of the vegetative states that we recognize as anger, tenderness, love, and hatred, but also the quite imperceptible drives to move, to say something, and to act in general. The mental processes become linked with the image of the body and the outside world through the actual experience of them. The brain is capable of a greater variety of patterns of situations than we actively employ; only those patterns become operative that the personal experience of self and the world have facilitated and made recurrent or potentially available. There is, therefore, no action that is purely mental, no thought without connection to reality. We can only mentally rearrange previous experience that is within our bodies, but then our rearrangements need not correspond with reality at all, and most of them do not, although the material is always borrowed from it.

Take for instance *right* or *left*. These are abstract notions. There is no right nor left that can be perceived without a body. And so the thought of right or left, having been formed of personal experience from and through the body, is part of that body. We think *right* and *left* by exciting the cortex patterns that were formed by the experience of right and left. The thought is the excitation of the pattern in the cortex while the rest of the cortex is inhibited; the overriding conscious control enables us to dissociate parts of patterns of previous experience from the whole. That this dissociation actually takes place, that the rest of the pattern of the previous experience is actually excited as part of the whole experience, can be demonstrated by the old well-known experiment of the pendulum. If you take any object in your hand, at the end of a string, that can serve as a pendulum, and if you remain completely still so as to damp out the oscillations of the pendulum, and then think *right* and *left* for a few seconds, the pendulum begins to oscillate from right to left. If you think *forward* and *back,* the oscillation will first become elliptic because of the inertia of the pendulum preserving its plane of oscillations, but in a few seconds the back and forward motion becomes quite clear. We see that the thought excites the muscles of the body, displacing the pendulum from right to left, or back to the rear and forward to the front. Although only partially, the inhibition comes from the thought *still,* and from our ability to dissociate particular items out of a whole situation—in this case, the dissociation of the nervous activity from the muscular. The greater our control of inhibition is, the more complete the dissociation is. If we direct ourselves to inhibition itself as a motive, we can gradually improve our control in this respect, too. Thus, if we think of the hand as *still,* and *right* and *left* as a new whole, the pendulum remains still while we think so. However, things may complicate themselves through (1) the phenomenon of *induction* and (2) the degree of skill previously acquired in inhibition control, as well as (3) the ability to project some thoughts while maintaining others as a canvas on which they all mix to become a plane situation.

The purely mental processes that are borne out by reality are possible only because they consist in rearranging patterns that were formed in some previous experience of the material self and world. Take, for instance, the act of reading, which is quite close to a purely mental activity, second only to thinking. Why do we need such a long time to read a page? We see it in one go; why do we not get the content at the same time? Largely because we have learned to read by pronouncing words, and this involves muscular action. We continue reading mentally word by word and cannot think faster than our muscles can work. As soon as this is realized, we can at once learn to read considerably faster by inhibiting the voiceless articulation of the words as they are scanned by the eyes. That is, when we dissociate the nervous activity from the whole situation of previous experience, our mental activity becomes more purely mental. Some even have defined thought as voiceless speaking. That may or may not be so; the important thing to us is that thought is a function formed through personal sensory and muscular activity.

Again, take the writing down of thoughts. Here we find the muscular activity slowing down and impeding thought. Now let us get rid of the actual writing. Just think and see yourself writing only mentally. We find again that we cannot see mentally the letters appearing in proper order and being properly formed much faster than by actually writing them down. There is even a method for teaching piano that consists of purely mental exercising to visualize touching the keys on the board without actually striking them. It is claimed that more rapid progress is achieved by this method than by the more usual ones. What interests us is that by speeding up muscular activity, we speed up thinking and *vice versa.* This obviously applies only to thoughts concerning action of the body.

It is easy to convince oneself by experience that thinking or mentally visualizing ourselves performing acts that we know we cannot do is practically impossible. It is as difficult to go mentally through any procedure as it is to perform it. For instance, the frigid woman who has never experienced orgasm, or the man who suffers from rapid and premature ejaculation, cannot think and follow through mentally a different procedure from the one known to them from their personal experience. They feel the same resistance in visualizing mentally a different performance from the habitual one as they do in practice, and the mental action is no more successful than the actual performance.

There seems to be an essential contradiction in all this; if we cannot think without a previous experience, and that experience is always an old manner of doing, how then is it possible to alter one's behavior to something more satisfactory? The answer is, "by learning"; that is, by forming a new pattern of body configuration and changing the material connected with the mental process. This is the same learning as when we learn to think in French by hearing and uttering French words, which with prolonged and methodical personal experience become more and more familiar until we can safely abandon our own language and finally completely stop translating it and begin to think directly in French. The absence of this direct active learning of the new manner of doing is the greatest drawback in present-day treatment. Freud believed that analysis is a method of teaching, as undoubtedly it is, when well done. But even then it does not make adequate use of direct active teaching, as it relies on the subject's tumbling to the better way after recognizing the faultiness of his own. The continuous refusal of the subject to abandon his position—the ingenious tricks of "resistance" to which he continually reverts as if he were fighting a battle in which he does everything to discourage his enemy (the analyst) from dislodging him from the spots he entrenched himself in for safety—is to a very large extent nothing more than the expression of the inability to give up English before one knows enough French. Only adequate knowledge of the new language can bring one to give up translating from one's mother tongue. Otherwise when rushed or taken unaware or when anything familiar is detected in the new situation, the old language is used before it is possible to do anything about it. Translated into emotional terms, the reversion to English could be said to be the resistance of the unconscious fighting its own battle.

In the early stages of learning, we are entirely concerned with linking up sensory perceptions with muscular activity, and with recognizing the situation by the emotional effect it produces in us. We learn to suck, to drink, to eat, to turn the head, to speak, to sit, and to stand, by facilitating some muscular pattern, and all the evidence of mental processes comes to us through voluntary muscular activity. Thoughts concerning realizable action are not any faster than the muscular action necessary to perform them. Every time we speak abstractly of the mind, ignoring its functional whole with the body and the external world, we reach conclusions that have little to do with reality. My contention is that learning always does involve the whole frame, and all learning that does not directly involve muscular activity is poor. The skill acquired otherwise can be used only when we are forewarned and have the leisure to think out every detail of the action beforehand. This will succeed only if nothing unforeseen occurs. In the actual performance, we soon find that we enact mostly what we have learned through muscular activity, in spite of all our labor to the contrary.

The basis of all learning is the reciprocity between mind and body, which is the conventional way of expressing the fact that the nervous system and the body are one whole organism. The experience of the body is necessary to form the linking of the nervous mechanisms with reality. Thereafter, the body is no longer essential, because the functioning of the nervous system and the electrochemical changes that go on in it can now be translated into terms of the external world, terms having objective meaning to all of us.

The next point on which clarity is necessary is how do we hope to influence the vegetative functioning of the body and to produce organic changes that are necessary if we essentially admit that there are voluntary and involuntary functions? The answer is that there is no difference in quality between the two sorts of functions, but simply a difference of degree. The voluntary muscles directly respond to our intention, the others only indirectly. So without knowledge and learning we cannot avail ourselves of their services, which seem then entirely autonomous. Let us examine some cases in detail.

The center constricting the bronchis is in the medulla oblongata. The inheritance and the previous personal history of this center determine its present state of sensitivity. In an asthmatic state this sensitivity is abnormally high and the bronchi are constricted spasmodically. We cannot at the moment regulate the bronchoconstrictor center directly by conscious inhibition. But we can affect the center indirectly; we can introduce into the body some antispasmodic drug, or we can exercise the conscious control that we have over our breathing. We can accelerate it, deepen it, or hold it. By doing so we do in fact influence the broncho-constricting center. Thus, by exercising the voluntary muscular control we affect the lower involuntary centers. By changing the breathing pattern we indirectly produce a change in the medulla, or at least something equivalent to it. There is compelling scientific evidence that the cerebrospinal and the vegetative organization of the body can be indirectly influenced by the voluntary motor centers to a much greater degree than we generally care to know.

On the occasion of Pavlov's centenary, Angus McPherson, reviewing the conditioned reflexes technique, cited numerous experiments, among which was the following: J. Hundgins* succeeded in giving a number of people voluntary control over their pupillary reaction, through which they learned to constrict or dilate their pupils at will. He first conditioned pupil constriction and dilation to the sound of a bell, by Casson's method; that is, by shining a strong light into the eyes at the sound of a bell. He then gave the patient a dynamometer. By squeezing the dynamometer at the command "Contract," the patient sounded the bell and shone the light on his own eyes. Then the patient was instructed to say in a whisper "Contract" or "Relax" while proceeding as before, then only say these words to himself while signaling as he did so. In the end, "the verbally controlled conditioned pupillary response had that appearance of spontaneity and control by the organism which are so characteristic of the behavior called voluntary."

There are numerous references in McPherson's paper to experiments conducted on similar lines where metabolic changes, visceral changes, and a host of all sorts of vegetative and reflex reactions have been organized for response in a desired way simply by conditioning; that is, by forming temporary connections between motor areas of the cortex and the lower centers of the nervous system.

---

*As reported in the *Journal of General Psychology* (March 8, 1933).

We often hear of patients absorbing some indifferent drug or even distilled water and obtaining the same results as if they absorbed a potent medicine, and we tend to ascribe the effect to their faith in the efficacy of the prescription or in the doctor. Paul Chauchard (in *Le Systeme Nerveux*, Presses Universitaires de France) refers to the following experiments: after injecting insulin (or some other active agent) for some time, one injects distilled water and obtains the same reduction of the sugar content of the blood as obtained after the insulin injection (or the effect corresponding to the other agent used). These experiments and results were obtained on mammals as well as men, so that there is no question of faith or autosuggestion, but only of the property of the cortex to initiate chain reactions in the lower centers once such reactions have been made the personal experience of the subject.

Professor J. H. Schultz of the Berlin University, the author of the autogen training method, has shown that with appropriate training we can dilate or constrict the blood vessels of any chosen point of the body. It is enough to think "My hand is warm," and the temperature of the hand rises a centigrade within a few seconds. Training oneself in special condition of relaxation, three times a day for one minute, enables one to achieve the immediate compliance of the blood vessels with the thinking of *warm* or *cold.* He has also trained his patients to contract and relax (for therapeutic purposes) the stomach, uterus, and other sphincter muscles.

We see, thus, that not only are the voluntary muscular mechanisms subject to our control, but the normally involuntary mechanisms and the vegetative functioning of the body are also subject to our control even though indirectly. Everybody knows that some people are masters of their emotions. We have already examined some of the mechanisms by which they have achieved that mastery. One of the most important mechanisms for directing action is inhibition and the associated phenomenon of induction. In order to obtain a monomotivated action, we must learn to inhibit the adjacent parasitic activity due to habit as well as the parasitic activity due to the topology of the cortex of the brain. If we could manipulate the nervous system itself, rearrange the nervous paths, and influence directly the different sources of impulses, we could probably obtain the wanted changes directly. As it is, we can learn to influence the nervous system by acting on its envelope. Mental processes are set going together with body action, and by the alternate switching of our attention from one plane to the other we obtain a unique mental motivation and feel the muscular sensation of such an act. It is through a series of such successive approximations that we can make sure of the correct use of the internal mechanisms of which we have no direct feeling or knowledge.

We have already insisted on the fact that the incompetent person is aware of imperfect adjustment in all of his functions, social, sexual, mental, and physical. As no act can be performed without the body's being directed by the nervous system, the habitual faulty self-management will also be used in learning any new mode of directing one's motivations. The new control must, therefore, be learned in conditions as remote as possible from any habitual act. By producing an entirely unfamiliar body pattern involving an unfamiliar muscular pattern, the breathing control and the sensation experienced are as different from the habitual ones as possible, so the reinstatement of habitual mental states has only a very remote chance of taking place. In these conditions we can learn to control inhibition and induction; in short, we learn to manage our motivation stock.

In the waking state, the background of all activity consists of the extensors—the muscles that extend the joints and elongate the body (also called "antigravity muscles" for that reason)—being tonically contracted by reflex impulses. When sitting or standing or doing anything at all, the extensors of the neck and of the lumbar region assume a habitual configuration, by which everybody recognizes us even from a distance. The manner of doing that is a personal characteristic is apparent in the body attitude even when we are doing as little as simply maintaining our space orientation without any special voluntary movement. The body-mind pattern involved has been learned and has grown with each of us for many years; it bears in it all the memories of our personal experience, that which is consciously remembered and that of which we are not aware.

The most complete elimination of the extensors in an act of spatial orientation would in fact be a complete contrast with our habitual experience and as little as possible associated with normal activity. Furthermore, the effort involved should be the smallest possible so that we can distinguish the slightest variations in muscular effort. For all sensations are so related to their causes that the slighter the cause, the smaller is the change that can be sensed. If we lift a heavy weight, for example, we cannot tell whether a sheet of paper is stuck beneath it or not. But on lifting a single sheet of paper we know at once if another one is stuck to it or not. Similarly, in daylight we do not notice a light bulb shining. But in the dark we can see the glow of a cigarette. Near an airplane, we cannot hear anything because of the propeller noise; in complete silence we can hear a fly or our own breath. Thus the intensity of the stimulus must be reduced if we want to become aware of small changes.

Lying on the back, head off the ground and the knees bent with the feet on the ground fulfills all these prerequisites. No extensor muscle is excited by gravitation acting on the nervous centers through habitual channels, and a minimum of muscular effort is necessary to maintain this attitude. Breathing is confined to abdominal movement, which is appropriate in this position.

But all this holds true only if there is no habitual faulty control. Otherwise the habitual excessive contraction of the extensors of the neck and the spinal extensors of the lumbar region is sensed as zero or no contraction, and the head cannot be brought into the normal position relative to the vertical. We sense strain and have to make an effort. The sensation of effort is due to the enaction of an antagonistic contraction of the muscles of the back of the neck, the extensors. In correct control, the two sets of muscles are antagonistic, and the contraction of the front ones would reflectively reduce the contraction in the back muscles that opposes the projected and enacted movement. In faulty con-

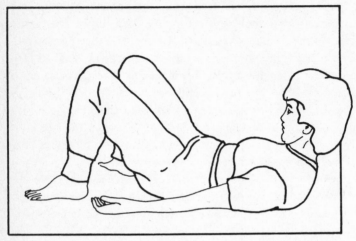

Lying on the back, head off the ground and knees bent.

trol, we have to force the front muscles to bring the head into the desired position and stretch those of the back of the neck which continue to contract. In correct control, bringing the head forward inhibits the muscles that oppose the movement. The thing to learn, therefore, is to improve the inhibition of the neck extensors. The neck extensors are voluntary muscles, and their contraction can only be due to habitually maintained contraction, which reaches zero level in the long run and goes beyond our inhibitory control. Maintaining the head raised for a prolonged time interval solves the difficulty. The phenomenon of induction thus becomes operative.

The strong excitation of any point of the cortex when prolonged or very intense tends to inhibit the surrounding area and *vice versa*—the inhibition of a point tends to excite the adjacent area. The reciprocal seesaw relationship of antagonistic groups of muscles is a particular case of induction. This phenomenon of induction has been used during the evolution of the species as a permanent fixture between muscles that are always called on to cooperate reciprocally while the time factor has gradually become reduced to nil. (Whether the course of evolution has actually followed this scheme is open to question, but it is a convenient formulation, enabling us to grasp different aspects of induction more readily.)

Maintaining the head raised for twenty or thirty seconds to begin with reduces the contraction of the back muscles of the head; these extensors become longer and allow the head to be lifted nearer to the normal vertical position. The actual amount of work done by the flexors decreases as the vertical component of the weight of the head increases and is borne by the cervical vertebrae. Thus, gravitation and physiology are acting as would be expected to adjust the action to that for which the human frame is fitted through the evolutionary adaptation of the frame to gravitation; the imperfect control tends to correct itself, and we act as does the properly adjusted person.

The person must now return to the initial lying position and learn what it feels like to act correctly. He must maintain this position over and over again, for at the beginning it is far from being correct. The important thing, however, is that the adjustment to the right response is produced by the internal mechanisms, precisely those in which the person had lost confidence. He found something sufficiently wrong with him to the extent of making him seek outside help, not knowing in fact that he already had all that was necessary to correct his adjustment to the external world.

After a few dozen trials, one becomes aware that the head lifting consists of two distinct movements, one of which is the movement of the support of the cranium; the other is the movement of the head around its support, which is seen when the chin is being lowered or lifted. By and by one learns to differentiate by feeling slighter and slighter differences in action and becomes able to command only the one for which there is motivation. At the same time, one becomes aware of the unrecognized motivation that is enacted by habit and that is, in the circumstances, parasitic and unwanted. One learns, therefore, what it feels like to produce a monomotivated act.

With the act becoming uniquely motivated, the sensation of effort disappears, and one becomes finally convinced through the sensation in his own body that resistance and effort are due to unrecognized motivation being enacted by the habit of presenting mixed or undifferentiated motivations, or even contradictory ones. Soon the act becomes completely reversible; that is, it can be halted at any moment, withheld, continued, or reversed without previous preparation.

The person should proceed slowly, remaining in the position described until an even and rhythmic breathing is obtained. As can be seen, even this apparently simple act of lying on the back with the head lifted off the ground is highly complex, and one needs time to sort out and realize what one is really doing. During that time, the physiological processes going on in the body assist in making the act correct. For one cannot maintain a physiologically incorrect position for any length of time without experiencing the sensation of effort as a new motivation; that is, an awareness of maintaining the position in spite of body tension contradicting it becomes operative.

When breathing becomes rhythmic and deep, the contraction around the mouth and in the fingers ceases. We have already seen that the alkalinity of the blood has some connection with muscular contraction. Thus, additional unwanted action, of which we are unaware because the habitual muscular contraction is too high to feel slight efforts, is cleared away. In many people the anal sphincter is also permanently fully contracted, and they can remedy this faulty action once the general tension is reduced.

Now a word of warning. The incompetent person, in whom dependence has brought about strong emotional disturbances, usually has at the back of his mind a nagging feeling of some impending doom, sin expiation, disaster, or deserved punishment. With such a disposition, he is inclined to attach mystical power to simple things. He may think, like a yogi, that special powers are attached to this position, in which he may feel for the first time the sense of well-being that one senses normally when no contradictory motivations are at work. Be aware that there is nothing in this position, except a convenient means of learning to recognize and direct some very normal processes.

The next thing to observe is that in order to lift the head something is produced in the lower abdomen. Put one hand on the lower abdomen very gently, and then lift your head. You will notice that the abdomen becomes "full" just before the head is lifted. The muscles that lift the head pull on both ends at which they are attached—at the head and the chest. In order to provide firm anchorage for the lower ends, the chest must be fixed to the bulk of the body weight. This anchoring is obtained by the abdominal muscles contracting and uniting the pelvis to the trunk. The state of the lower abdomen, which does not interfere with breathing yet feels full, is the correct state and is the condition in which it is normally found at the moment of correct action.

Nor is this all that we can learn from this simple act. If you put one hand at the small of your back, you perceive that on lifting your head to the normal position in space the small of the back straightens and fills up the space that is formed by the lumbar curve of the spine when the head is on the ground and the legs stretched.

Thus it becomes quite clear that the pelvic bone is a primary mover in anything we do. The head rests on the cervical vertebrae, which make up a flexible rod capable of bending in all directions and rotating or twisting around itself. The trunk as a whole rests on a similar rod formed by the lumbar vertebrae. Rotation (and twisting) of the body can be done smoothly and simply only if these two rods are fully used. The lower end of the lumbar rod must be fixed in any new position before it is capable of receiving the weight on the upper end. The same is true of the cervical rod carrying the head.

All correct action starts with the movement of the pelvic bone, which displaces itself so as to carry the spine and the head through to the new position while allowing the head complete freedom of movement. The control of the head and of the pelvic bone are, therefore, absolutely essential to all correct action. One is not more important than the other. Both must be controlled correctly to obtain correct action. In some acts the position of the head is more telling and easier to notice, but it cannot be obtained without proper control of the pelvis. As far as the sexual act is concerned, the complete mobility of the pelvis is essential. The case of the physically handicapped is treated in my book *Higher Judo.* * Most people seem to have both stiff necks and stiff hips, yet they have managed apparently to live a satisfactory life (see my book *Body and Mature Behavior*).† The answer is that such people are adjusted to a definite set of conditions and go completely out of gear in sharply changed environmental conditions. They can manage only in conditions that allow them to think through the planned movement before acting, or during the repetition of familiar actions.

The reader will also find in *Body and Mature Behavior* a full explanation of how anxiety is gradually abated in this position on the back. The explanation is not necessary, of course, in order to sense the effect, because the effect is not achieved by suggestion, but by a physiological phenomenon connected with parasympathetic and sympathetic balance (discussed later on).

The next step in learning correct action is in the simplest movement of sitting up from the lying on the back position. This is one of the earliest movements of the entire body that a child learns. The first way a child sits up consists generally in pressing the back of the head against the ground or bed, lifting and twisting the hips so as to bring both knees onto the ground. The child then disengages the shoulder and rests the forehead on the ground, and now is in a position to support the body on all fours and finally to sit up. Without supervision or a sufficient number of illustrations, it is rather difficult to get this movement right.

But it is not really important to copy nature in detail in order to learn correct control. We may, therefore, start with the next way

---

*Groundwork *(Katemewaza)*, vol. I of *Higher Judo* (London: Warne, 1942).
†(London: Routledge and Kegen Paul, 1949).

of getting up, because we already have the muscular capacity for any movement, whereas the child is compelled to follow a certain course.

Lie on your back as usual, and lift your head to its normal position in space. Make sure that there is no stiffness in the neck muscles, by scanning the horizon with your eyes and feeling your head following without strain or change in the breath rhythm. Then lift both feet off the ground and flex your thighs, bringing both knees over your lower abdomen. Remain in that position until you feel your breath becoming even again. Now put your feet back on the ground and lift your knees once more, making sure that you do not hold your breath and that there is no resistance; that there is no unnecessary contraction and that the movement is completely reversible (can be stopped at any instant and reversed smoothly).

Repeat this several times. Now put your hand on your lower abdomen and try again. Observe the fullness of the lower abdomen when the movement conforms with all the requirements of correct action. Now move your hands as if to push your knees

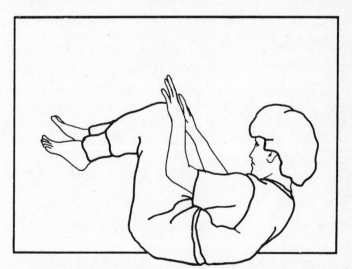

Move your hands as if to push your knees away from you.

away from you, while maintaining the abdomen in the same state. Note that in order to sit up without effort, without holding your breath, with the movement remaining reversible all the way through, your chin moves against your throat very slightly. This pressure is necessary if the atlas is to support the head by compression only. Before repeating, reset your abdominal state—not stiff, but full—and sit up. The sitting up should now feel in performance very graceful and pleasurable, and the whole movement looks and feels like one simple, continuous act. The word *continous* needs to be understood in its mathematical sense; that is, the velocity of all the vertebrae of the body in movement varying gradually (the hodograph presenting no point of inflection), the angular velocity of every point from the pelvis upward being the same at every instant.

Proceed very slowly, and take as long as necessary, until you are sure that your feeling corresponds to reality; that is, that other people can recognize in your movements all the mentioned points of importance. You then know how it feels to act correctly. With this gauge, proceed to learn how to get up onto your feet, to stand, to speak, eat, make love, work, excrete, and think. In practice, it is expedient to proceed under guidance for a longer period; in total about thirty lessons are sufficient for the average person. But he learns nothing really new. All that happens is that the student gets a clearer and keener sensation of correct action. The student is also helped by the induction method described in my book *Body and Mature Behaviour* and by other refinements of technique to restore the full range of flexibility of all articulations, in particular the full mobility of the hip joints and the head. The intelligent reader should be able to rediscover these means guided solely by the feeling of correct action. The task is not an easy one, but it is also not impossible.

VOLITION AND MUSCULAR TENSION

Everybody knows the feeling of seizure that is experienced when the whole musculature is violently contracted, as in the face of unexpected and fatal danger. Standing on top of a high building and just contemplating jumping over to the adjacent one, even only a few feet away, one can feel quite clearly the onset of generalized contraction of the musculature. In this state of high-level contraction it is impossible to make oneself jump—nor is it possible to make one obey any orders in this state. If the jump is to save one from an even greater danger, the jump may be attempted, but if the tension is not relieved in time and the jump attempted with the utmost will effort, it is unlikely to be successful.

In the state of generalized complete contraction of the musculature, one is impervious to suggestion. In violent rage or anger, one is completely refractory to any suggestion from without or within oneself.

In the state of hypnosis, one also loses entirely the ability to command oneself, but is at the highest state of involuntary suggestibility. Before this state of suggestibility is obtained, complete relaxation of the musculature must be achieved. Moreover, as Professor J. H. Schultz has shown, the relaxation must be extended so far as to relax the capillaries and the small blood vessels. The muscular relaxation coincides with the sensation of heaviness in the limbs and in the body, and the dilation of the blood vessels coincides with the sensation of warmth. In such complete relaxation, the person is in the most suggestible state. It is not necessary to lose consciousness to reach this state of complete suggestibility. In the state of complete muscular and vascular relaxation, without any loss of consciousness, one is open to suggestion both from without and within oneself.

In the state of complete contraction, one loses completely the sense of weight of the body and limbs. Between these two extreme states—complete contraction and complete passive relaxation—is a continuous scale, the middle of which is the state where the voluntary contractions are absent and the body is held in tonic contraction, which coincides with a sensation of lightness and unity of the body. In this state, suggestibility is greater than in complete contraction and lesser than in complete relaxation. It is the optimum state for learning; that is, for acquiring new responses. New experience in this state enjoys greater transference; the learning is transferred to adjacent patterns more readily than in the state of contraction, and self-control is easier.

The state of suggestibility is also the state of passivity. The entire musculature is relaxed, the vessels are relaxed, the body is heavy and warm, and there is no incentive to do anything. In the tonic state, however, the muscles are not flabby and not contracted. The body feels light, the vessels neither dilate nor constrict, the body is not warm or cold, but just cool. The entire frame is tuned up not for violent efforts, but for smooth, easy action such as clear thinking, dancing, or pirouetting. These states have obviously much to do with the sympathetic and parasympathetic balance. The excitation of the sympathetic system obtains in the state of self-assertion, as in fighting or producing violent efforts. The parasympathetic brings about restfulness and fosters the recuperative functions.

In the state of complete relaxation, self-assertiveness is reduced, being incompatible with complete passive suggestibility. It is, therefore, possible to produce useful changes in oneself. However, in complete relaxation the level of self-assertiveness is too low for actively learning new modes of action. The tonic state is more appropriate for normal active self-direction. The habitual long-standing contractions are in sufficient contrast with the general sensation of lightness to be detected readily, yet one is in active normal positions and not in the state of inactivity as in complete relaxation.

It is impossible to achieve tonic *acture* straight away. Only by gradually learning can one learn to inhibit the unwanted contractions and—by using reciprocal innervation and the inductive properties of reciprocal functions—can one achieve true tonic posture or *acture.*

14. First General Overhaul

After four or five lessons, note that the head comes more easily to the normal position, the eye axis becomes horizontal, and the position can be held for two or even three minutes without strain. The breathing becomes even and deep due to the entire mobilization of the abdomen and chest. A sense of ease and repose pervades the whole body. Soon the muscles around the mouth and the muscles of the fingers, especially the thumb, lose their tenseness and feel light. This is the first inkling of the feeling of the body in a state of monoactivation and monomotivation. Only some grossly unnecessary contractions are as yet removed; nevertheless, the sensation is sufficiently clear to be recognized.

While the flexors are contracted, the extensors elongate. When standing, therefore, your posture is more erect thanks to the latent effect of the stretch reflex and nervous induction (see *Body and Mature Behavior*). Posture is thus corrected by the same internal mechanisms as in good carriage, not by an act of volition (which fails every time your attention is shifted).

Having learned to recognize the posture that produces the feeling of enacting a clear motivation, it is possible to extend the skill to other planes of activity. Generally one also becomes aware of the motive for the muscle contraction when one feels them decontracting. Some very gross contramotivations suddenly stand out clearly, and if they are not particularly strongly sustained by the environment at the present moment, it is even possible to get rid of them at once.

And if there is no spontaneous realization of the parasitic motivation, it is enough to think of the particular part of the body in which decontraction is sensed to become aware of it. In this way, a rough first general overhaul of attitude and sensation becomes possible even at this stage.

After a few minutes of proper ventilation of the lungs, the muscles of the mouth relax. Food intake is very often linked with extraneous motivation. Some eat all their lives in order to become "strong boys or girls," and not because there is any special body tension requiring food intake. Some eat with a vague feeling of economic insecurity or social standing nagging at the back of their minds. Some eat mainly to dull the sensation of impotence. The place, the manner of mastication, the sitting attitude, the breathing are all affected by and have a decisive influence on digestion. Either the person acts out of a sense of duty and forces herself to get on with something she really does not want to do, or she proceeds to stuff herself for the purpose of feeling the heavy sensation of an overfull stomach. Her breathing is arrhythmic, and every mouthful requires attention. These faults can now be corrected.

It is difficult to enumerate all the infinite varieties of improper eating. But they all have this in common: a motivation having nothing to do with release of the tension called hunger is enacted at the same time by habit and makes eating a source of emotional disturbance. The person generally sticks to a diet no one could maintain for any length of time without stirring up similar digestive trouble. The alkalinity of the blood is partially neutralized by excessive acidity of the digestive tracts. Pains, indigestion, nausea, constipation, or diarrhea follow. Each one of these complaints fit a particular habitual pattern of cross motivation.

People with long intestinal tracts, who have long bodies and short legs, misled to use a rich meat or protein diet suffer as much as those with short intestinal tracts who are vegetarians. In all cases of misdirection of oneself, strong emotional motivation is grafted onto the essential motive of food intake. There are people who drink excessively at meals, not because they are thirsty, but because they think it is "good" for them. As we have very weak feeding instincts, we have no means of resisting any of the emotional parasitic motivations that ruin us by creating bad feeding habits.

Both regularity and irregularity are often exaggerated by habitual motivations that should have nothing to do with feeding. The reader should now be able to recognize the most obvious ones, not by a knowledge of food chemistry and the physiology of digestion, but by the feelings of resistance, irreversibility, and halted breath that present themselves in all acts improperly motivated.

This first examination is important not only because of physical health, but also because the same kind of thing is involved in the sexual behavior of the incompetent as it is in all that she does. Often the feeling of discomfort due to digestive trouble is mistaken for sexual trouble. The reason for this is that the all-important security-dependence pattern has distorted the emotional texture, and has so mixed up motivation that the person's action does not relieve the tension that is present, but corresponds to another one that she is unable to recognize. She habitually mistakes the desire for approval, affection, security, for sexual desire and finds herself frigid not because she has no sexual potency, but in fact, because her direction of self prevents parasympathetic dominance —so there *is* no sexual tension to be released.

With the increased ability of recognizing extraneous contractions, one might, even at this stage, be able to notice at the end of a lesson, when breathing has become very regular and easy, that the anal sphincter is often habitually contracted. Men usually find that they can maintain or boost up a failing erection by contracting the anal sphincter. Normally they do not really know what they are doing, but they are satisfied with a vague sensation of effort. Thus, while holding their breath and listening to themselves they are afraid to do anything at all in case they interfere with the appearance of an erection. The anxious expectation and the contracted anal sphincter interfere with the building up of the sexual tension that needs complete freedom from any voluntary interference in the state of contraction of the pelvic floor and the skeletal muscles.

By recognizing the presence or the absence of contraction in the anal sphincter, it is possible to discover the extraneous motive for its contraction. Once the lower pelvic floor is freed from this improper habitual stiffening of the anal sphincter, greater freedom of movement of the pelvis becomes possible.

Although this overhaul is only a rough examination of one's

improper control and does not remove the reasons for it, the realization that one actually does enact that something that brings about the sensation of resistance and anxiety accompanying the sexual act brings great relief. Prior to this realization, one felt punishment, abandonment, or other disaster impending. So the general tension of the body increased to the point of producing perspiration, palpitation, diarrhea, flatulence, or whatever other personal form it took. There was no apparent reason for all these phenomena, and one had to accept that there was something somewhere fundamentally wrong and the hour of reckoning was imminent. With the building up of the ability to recognize cross motivation, one can sense that the tenseness and anxiety are due to something that one actually enacts and something that one knows now how to better deal with. Thus the feeling of guilt or shame fades away. Quite often people with sufficient training in clear thinking feel their mistaken action so distinctly that they are able to change their environment sufficiently to eliminate the habitual faulty response without any further learning. There is no need for absolute perfection; it is enough to be able to follow the task in hand without being distracted by sensing a constant, nagging, but unrecognized motivation. Further progress is assured by learning to place oneself into more appropriate environmental conditions and hence to join greater flexibility of attitude and response in adverse ones.

Do not try to correct your faults by an effort of will. When we make such efforts, we feel the resistance that is due to extraneous unrecognized motivation. We are therefore exercising and improving resistance at the same time, although not to the same degree. A lot of energy and perseverence are necessary before the difference will become marked enough to satisfy. Wait until you have learned to bring your body and mind to a state in which it is more easily controlled and is more capable of enacting any clear motivations that are presented. This state will come about when you have learned to control the sympathetic-parasympathetic balance.

15. About the Technique

The whole man must move at once. The inability to do so is lifted when the contradictory motivations are lifted; this coincides with relieving the contractions enacted with or without awareness. To make this possible in all situations, we must learn to bring ourselves into the state of potency in which we can enact what we wish correctly. There are innumerable methods of achieving this. It is only a question of which method is the most appropriate and most expedient in each case. We have seen that environment, mind, and body are an indivisible one. No method is effective that deals with any one of these alone. The paradoxical situation of improvement being obtained either by psychological or physical treatment is resolved when we realize that methods that seem to deal with mind alone or body alone do in fact deal with the person as a whole—whether they admit it or not. The question is only "Which part of the whole situation is attacked more directly?" If in each situation the whole frame is dealt with directly, it is much easier to bring about the desired result.

The important thing to realize is not that we can deal effectively with, say, a duodenal ulcer by surgical intervention or by psychological treatment, but that we must do so by addressing the functional unity of environment, mind, and body. This unity seems to be a stumbling block to all of us, as the body-mind concept is an abstraction that grew into our language and understanding. Most people will agree that the body and the mind are two aspects of the same thing, or two poles of the same entity, but they still cannot appreciate that there is no mind without environment. Ignore the personal experience of the environment of the nervous system—that is, the body and the external world—and there is nothing left that recalls mental life at all. Thoughts or feelings without their actual content due to the personal experience of the environment are nothing more than electrical changes in the structure of the nervous system. It is the connection of these changes with the environment that makes such a change into a feeling of affection for somebody, or into a sensation of red, or into the ideas of continuity, acceleration, beauty, or justice.

Let us examine the functional unity of the example just mentioned. Not everybody can give himself an ulcer by justified or imaginary worry. One must first learn to become an "ulcerous" person before worry will enable him to get an ulcer. The individual history of a nervous system, its hereditary environment, the actual physical environment, and the social medium form a person's attitude and reactions to events—in short, they form character. It is the person's own history that has formed his attitude to his mistakes and to those of others, his carriage, his ways of eating and overloading his stomach, his compulsive being on time, his exacting the same machinelike precision from those surrounding him, his compulsive needing to have things just right, his neurotic trend to perfection, his inability to cope with failure, and his demands on his wife, his children, his subordinates and superiors—to say nothing of his sexual life, which is certainly not irrelevant in this connection.

This man's adjustment to the environment has formed such an *acture* that he feels right only when reacting with heightened emotional tone to anything that is important to him. Adrenalin secretion is increased, muscular tension augmented at every action; in short, worry and anxiety underlie all functioning. Even his happiness and merrymaking are tinted with worry: he cannot laugh heartily, but only smile; all his *acture* is unspontaneous.

At a certain stage the ulcer is simply his most striking symptom of an ulcerous behavior adjustment and has reached a stage where an operation is the urgent intervention that will save him. But an operation is far from being purely a body affair. To have to lie down and let somebody play with a knife in one's insides is an emotional experience equivalent to an abreaction on the analyst's couch. A person who has some sense may benefit by this experience and begin to think and to see things in their true perspective. He may realize the futility of hurrying for its own sake, for there he is pinned to his bed, yet the world continues spinning round just as if nothing at all had happened. He may get an insight into his own insignificance in the general scheme of things, and his unique importance to himself and to those who depend on him. In short, maturity may suddenly catch up with him, and he will get up a new man.

Moreover, together with all of that is the anesthetic shock, the fact that he cannot move, and the fact that his food is being regulated by somebody who is rational about it. For several weeks he will be prevented from indulging in all those habits that are the real complex of his complaint. A surgical intervention is an emotional experience and a lesson whether we want it or not. If learning has taken place, there is a psychosomatic change and success is assured. On the other hand, if the only thing that has happened is the removal of some tissue, although a corresponding local improvement will occur, we will soon be meeting the same ulcerous bore as before, but now with a properly sewn-up stomach.

Similarly, a psychologist's treatment may be a purely psychic affair with only minor effects, or it may be a full environmental, psychosomatic, emotional experience with a corresponding change of *acture.* In the presence of a skilled and objective analyst, the patient breathes differently, and breathing has a lot more to do with the alkalinity of the blood than is commonly appreciated. This improved breathing reduces the patient's compulsiveness, and the reduced general emotional tone may produce a marked change in muscular tension, so that postural improvement will follow. He may even stop bolting his food. Again, the improvement will be proportional to the psychosomatic environmental reform. Otherwise, there will be a lot of knowledge uncovered about Oedipal, castration, and other complexes, with some minor removal of symptoms, but just before the final triumph of the analyst over his invisible opponent, the unconscious—the wicked, ungentlemanly unconscious—in a last desperate effort of "resistance" will win the battle by producing a hemorrhage. For the "unconscious," as everybody knows by now, prefers the surgeon to the analyst.

We can see that any method may solve the problem, depending on what the subject makes of it. The merit of a method, however, depends only on what it does directly. The integration, or transfer of learning, of the directly brought-about change into the intimate *acture* of the person depends on the patient's ability to learn. With this rule in mind, we can understand that improving the learning ability of the person is the real foundation of good *acture* and therefore the foundation for the good health of (what cannot be said otherwise) the "mind-and-body." From this standpoint, it is obvious that improvement should be directed to what is common to all action; that is, to the fundamental properties of the nervous system, excitation, inhibition, induction, and so on, which are the conscious mind's means of control over the functioning of the whole system. If we can produce a more harmonious functioning of the frame through learning to control motivation, inhibition, and induction, we can achieve that mastery over self that is the essence of conscious life.

The major reason why we start with the body is as follows. When we do something or cannot do something, we experience a certain state that is very familiar to each of us, but that is quite different for every one of us. The personal language in this state is sensory and kinesthetic, and therefore it is very difficult to translate into a spoken language having a common meaning. What you mean by *easy, love,* or *gentle,* is not the same as what I mean when using such words. The nearest way in which we can translate subjective experience is by using symbolism. "I feel like flying," or "like sinking," or "like bursting" are all symbolic expressions of subjective sensations.

One of the great achievements of Freud was his method of breaking through this barrier of personal symbolism by interpreting the subjective personal language to the patient himself, thus making him aware of the real motives behind his action. By acting on the body directly (as when asking a person to assume a given position or make a precise movement), it is possible to avoid the laborious, lengthy, and often faulty translation from personal language into words and *vice versa.* We no longer need to find out the rational interpretation of the body sensations; neither do we need to make sure that the spoken words will be correctly translated by the person into his own subjective language. This direct teaching of the person to understand subjectively the correct meaning of his sensations makes him see in his motivation more than he is normally aware of. The awareness of motivation is necessary before the person can learn a new management of motivation and thus change his behavior. Freud considered analysis not as an operation of sorting out motivations from one another, but as a teaching method for managing isolated motivations.

The present technique is mainly concerned with learning a better mode of action and uses the body, from which the person can learn directly, in his own body language. The usual resistance is avoided, as the person is learning to feel resistance in himself in matters that do not intensely compromise his emotional security, and is thus given the means of dissolving it. It goes without saying that this technique is not the best in all cases. Shortcuts are not applicable where the disintegration of personality is too deep and reeducation cannot be left in the hands of the person himself. Such people are not able to apply themselves to the arduous task of learning without expert guidance, and so other methods must be used. However, the majority of people who seek improvement on their own initiative are fit to take care of themselves and should find in this technique enough to satisfy them.

The main feature of the technique consists in making available the full range of functioning in all planes, the idea behind it being *not* that spontaneity is enacting any wild urge that happens to exist, but that *all* action is spontaneous when it is not compulsive. This formulation sounds evasive, but only at first, for compulsion is a positive parasitic addition. When in control of the full range of voice production, one uses the pitch and intonation that is appropriate or expedient and feels no compulsion about it. If one can produce only one pitch, that may be satisfactory in most circumstances, but there are always circumstances in which the habitual manner is inadequate. If no other means are available the habitual and appropriate manner becomes compulsive for lack of range or alternative. The compulsive *acture* is not bad in itself; it becomes compulsive only because it is enacted out of place, in a manner in which it was enacted in previous experience when it was fitting. The person—being unable to dissociate previous experience—is enacting past experience now, as an automaton responds to all experience by setting off with the same response.

The person with the rigid moral code adhered to by compulsion, for lack of mastery of self-control, is like the man who is erect because he cannot bend his spine. Just as a healthy spine is capable of an infinite variety of configurations and, therefore, remains properly curved (even when held stiff, if necessary), so the moral code should be flexible and usable in both extremes of polarity. Only then can we accept restraint without revolt and compulsion; we achieve the freedom of necessity. The person who never refuses anybody because he cannot may seem kind, but is most of the time suffering from his own goodness. He does more harm in his own charming manner to himself and to others than do healthy people who are good when necessary and cruel when it is justified. It is as if using a knife to cut living flesh were a bad thing in itself, and, therefore, surgery is a wicked profession.

The inability to do is almost without exception due to compulsive fixity of the function in question to only one rung of the ladder of function, all the others being excluded. Action interests the large parts of the cortex, and areas that are constantly inhibited interfere with all action. Impotence is not a local inability, but a general failure of *acture.*

We, therefore, do not teach The Correct Way to Breathe, but all possible modes of breathing. We do not teach people to hold the stomach drawn up and flat, but the full range of abdominal contraction, from blown-out expansion to complete emptiness of the abdominal cavity, such as practiced in yoga. The same holds true for the pelvis, the head, and every joint of the body. The end effect is that in each situation the frame adjusts itself in the best possible way, because we become aware of parasitic contractions maintained for no purpose but by dint of corrupt *acture* alone. The full range of inhibition and excitation is thus explored, and the person becomes capable of conscious action and of assuming full responsibility for it.

There is practically no connection between this method of reeducation of the frame and gymnastics. We do not achieve the full range of play of each articulation by repetition, muscle exercising, or increasing speed and force, but by widening and refining the cerebral control of the muscular range. All we do is done very slowly. All difficulty in performance is relieved not by making strenuous efforts with willpower and force to achieve the projected act, but by using induction to make the faulty control perceptible. Thus, contradictory action is lifted by recovering the ability to inhibit the contracted parts and excite the flabby, toneless ones. It is not rare to reestablish the full range of an articulation in a few minutes, while simple exercising would take months to do so. Moreover, the subject learns the *art* of learning, which is applicable to all function. And the gained control, once integrated into normal behavior, remains effective without any special attention and exercising of the articulation.

Here are a few practical examples. The object in exploring a fuller range of spinal flexion is to learn what it feels like to reduce the contraction of the extensors. From the original lying position, lift your legs and hips off the ground and rest your weight on the shoulders, motionless, in the most comfortable way you can do this. The variety of possible configurations is quite wide. Observe your attitude for the purpose of comparison with the one you will assume spontaneously later on. Free the lower abdomen from unnecessary tension, and let your breath take its own rhythm. So long as there is stiffness in your body due to holding the breath, not only is the latter audible and aperiodic, but the legs will remain fixed in space. As soon as your personal rhythm of breathing is allowed to continue (which means inhibiting all unnecessary contractions), the legs will oscillate gently in synchronism with the

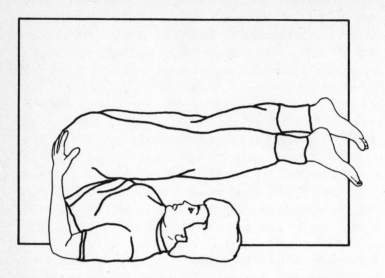

Lift your legs and hips off the ground and rest your weight on your shoulders.

breath. Remaining in this position for about a minute and thinking of even breathing does the trick. Even breath is established. Possibly the parasitic stiffening is due to the motivation of being stiff, or perhaps the idea that one is old, or a fear of weakness in the neck muscles (which creates the body sensation of danger to the neck), or to whatever other motivation you may discover. Simply inhibiting the extraneous motivation by clearly projecting the idea of freedom from strain produces in a few seconds a further curving of the spine; it is not rare to suddenly find the personal motive behind the hitherto unrecognized stiffness. Now the legs move toward the head with every expiration when the curvature of the spine increases, and move away from the head with every inhalation. This means that inhalation is being produced by tensing the extensors of the back, and a further lengthening of these is possible in everyone, as indeed they produce it in every expiration.

A further reduction of the contraction of the back muscles in this position is obtained by putting your hands on your knees and then pressing the knees against the hands. This pressure should be mild and kept up for ten to twenty seconds without remission. This continuous contraction of the flexors of the hips and the abdomen, maintained without interfering with the breath, further lowers the contraction of the back extensors. Hold your hands on your knees in whatever position of body flexion you can without strain.

Some backs are vertical, while other backs are rounded and inclined to the vertical. The first have the body resting on the neck line of the shoulders, while the others have the shoulderblades on the ground. In either of these cases, it is possible to lift the head off the ground, especially when helping yourself gently with your hands to raise the head. Obviously, then, a further rolling back

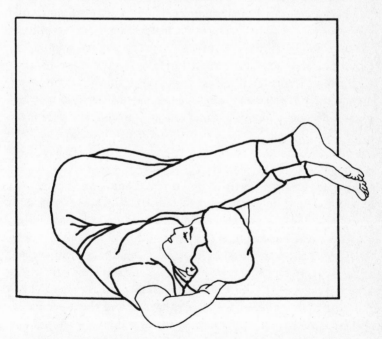

Lift the head off the ground, especially when helping gently with the hands.

and bringing the feet well over your head is not hindered by anything else but the stiffening of the shoulder and neck joints. It is enough to hold the breath, as when expecting pain or danger, to produce the stiffening of the neck and shoulders. By learning to inhibit this parasitic motivation, the body rolls over still further.

You can further fold up your body by touching the ground with one foot—say, the right one—well to the right of the head, and the other one well to the left. After exploring the ground with your feet, you can touch every point on a wide arc of a circle and bring both feet together just above your head.

The sensation of the body is now to be memorized. Simply by reinstating the memorized sensation or body image, once the body is straightened into the lying position, you can bring it back to complete folding with your feet touching the ground above your head. By clearly projecting the mental image of the body free from interfering contractions all along the spine, it is possible to fold over so as to touch the floor with the insteps. Those whose attitude is "I am no good" or "It is difficult" or "This needs training" or "I am too old," etc., are invited to lift or bypass these parasitic motivations by maintaining only those directions that are necessary to the projected act. Many people succeed beyond their expectations and within only three or four lessons, especially if the same muscular groups are attacked in different positions and the transfer of learning is directed actively. In these cases success is quite general.

Now get up very slowly, without strain and, after a minute or so, observe and note the effect of induction on the extensors of your back. These muscles, having been inhibited for a considerable time, now become tonically alive and tend to raise the body to the correctly toned posture. You now stand taller without any voluntary self-direction to do so; moreover, your habitual carriage now feels awkward. Nevertheless, revert to it so that you can learn how the more correct posture feels better, and therefore realize that by exploring the full range of the function you will tend to choose the better over the less satisfactory; the better posture is the one found and maintained not by lack of alternatives, but by widened range of ability.

More is learned in this lesson than is immediately apparent. Control of mental direction is improving, and one learns the importance of clear thinking, while allowing the projected action to be enacted. The learning is done in one's own body language; weeks of verbal interchange may not achieve so intimate a recognition of the fact that the inability to do is due to voluntary projection of parasitic habitual patterns, of which one can become aware when the level of excitation is reduced. When the tension present is small, the kinesthetic sense is refined and becomes capable of detecting smaller and smaller differences. But perhaps the most interesting feature of this lesson is that one discovers that one's own resources are not only not fully used, but are actively prevented from being used.

To bring a person to realize emotionally that what happens to him is the result of his misuse of himself, that he uses an infantile emotional pattern without awareness, one has to break through his resistance to the analyst by giving timely interpretations of his behaviors and attitudes. Here the breaking of the resistance is done directly, in the most intimately understood body language; the person is not asked to give up the old pattern, which he cannot do, before he has another substitute. By enlarging his range of ability, he gains freedom of choice, and the compulsiveness attached to a unique alternative is lifted. The ability to do abrogates the old, impotent *acture* by the same mechanism with which we reject all action that does not open the door and choose the one that does. One is not reluctant to give up action that does not work properly when in possession of a correct method that does so; one even feels somewhat foolish for not having thought of it before.

The interpersonally trifling importance of the action of flexing the body (for indeed, what does it matter whether one's body is flexible or not?) has, nevertheless, a much deeper internal personal significance. The importance of any act is derived from its social value, *but* from the point of view of internal functioning the exclusion of physiological action to the point of inability to use it is of immense importance. The *acture* of a person is the same whether he tries to flex his body, solve an important social problem, or empty his bowels. The way he mobilizes himself for anything is a personal constant that changes only very slowly unless directly attacked.

Thus, an experienced teacher can detect a great variety of extraneous motivations that interfere with the accomplishment of complete flexion even in these first static states of *acture*. He can note that Mrs. X keeps her knees together even when she loses her balance, where the reflective righting response would normally bring one leg away from the other in order to regain equilibrium. He may be sure that Mrs. X's attitude toward sex is not free from shame or some other motivation that is beyond her control. He can see that the other person (Mr. G) is constantly aware of his anus, and will probably find later on that hemorrhoids and constipation play an important part in Mr. G's emotional makeup. With experience, the teacher is able to detect the part of the body that is in the person's mental self-image, more or less permanently, and produces parasitic contractions in every action.

However, it does no good to mention these findings; to do so would only provoke a flood of rationalizations, which are necessary to sustain the personal *acture;* they constitute what analysts call *resistance.* Our way is to first give the student the means to act without bringing into action his habitual self-mobilization. Once he is in command of a fuller range of action in the particular function, the habitual manner (in which resistance is part of the adjustment and without which the person cannot act at all) is resolved. Compulsiveness is lifted in that particular function, because of the available alternative mode. At this juncture, the resistance becomes quite conscious, often as sudden insight or what is known as *satori* in zen practice.

Resistance is resolved through becoming unnecessary. The sudden insight that results is then charged with only moderate affect, and does not present the danger that premature interpretation does in analytic practice. Later on we will give some examples of sudden insights.

There are many other advantages in this position where the body is nearly inverted in the gravitational field. The blood supply to the head is increased for several minutes on end. Once the forced dilation is over, the dilated vessels contract and the head feels cool, as in the state of proper self-control. In most languages there is an idiomatic expression connecting the sensation of coolness of the head (or, more vaguely, of the blood) to denote the state of potent self-control: "cool-headed," *avec sang froid, chladnokrovno, kaltblutig,* and *bkorrauch.* Also, the breathing is now produced by the soft abdominal content *pressing* to expel air, instead of the usual pulling. Moreover, rest of the normally working centers and the induction effect afterwards brings new tone into them.

The next step after having explored a fuller range of a function (in this case, the flexion of the spine) is to learn reversibility. Reversibility is to dynamics of body action what unstable equilibrium is to static states. Attention is to be focused now on the way of directing oneself in action. The dynamics of an act change very considerably with the body image of the person. Thus, the person may act with his feet being in the limelight of his attention. The feet at once become contracted and play the leading part in the action. The rest of the body adjusts itself so that the feet may follow exactly the trajectory that is mentally projected as a goal to be achieved.

Note that not only the geometrical trajectory is directed, but the velocity all along the trajectory, and the changes of velocity—in short, the rhythms—are sensed simultaneously with the act. The learning consists in acquiring the ability of projecting the movement and following it through in space, projecting the kinesthetic sensations before the act, and then enacting the mental-body image of the sensation in actual performance. For example, the head may be sensed, as the location so to speak, of the "I," and the head is at once held fixed. The person's mental eye is focused on the kinesthetic sensations in the region of the head; the rest of the body is auxiliary and is used so as not to interfere with the head's trajectory. It is impossible to explain in words exactly what is meant by feeling the "I" here or there, without sounding mystical or even less rational. The difficulty is the same as in trying to translate into verbal language any internal sensation. The only way is to experience bodily the same thing, and to make some symbol as a label for identifying it (so let us better proceed with experimenting).

Now, from the usual lying on your back position, roll your body directly into the final position, with your feet touching the ground overhead. Most people hold their breath, turn red in the face, and feel considerable effort. To find a better way, one must learn to mentally project the action without interfering with the breath, without stiffening the neck or fixing the head in any way—in short, without doing anything that is not related to the act. Now this is seemingly an arduous task, for one has to learn to integrate a considerable number of acts into one unique complex act. This is the erroneous element, introduced into action by ignorance, which makes training, training, and yet more training necessary. By actively learning what is being transferred from "training," it is possible to cut out most of the futile labor. By exploring the full range of the action in space and in time with the gauge of reversibility as the indicator of what to refuse, one obtains all the advantages of trial-and-error learning as well as the added clarity of monomotivation.

The reversibility check consists in experiencing that the *acture* of the body is made such that action can be stopped all along the procedure and reversed without any preparation. This enables a person to bring about in himself an unfamiliar configuration and state of direction, and maintain it throughout the act. The body experience is the essential thing for realizing what reversibility is; no amount of understanding can convey more than a very rough mental substitute.

All the time required must be allowed for everyone to experiment with himself. The better way of doing must be arrived at by personal choice. The correct manner of doing must have no moral compulsion of being "right" because it is from another authority; one's own consent must be obtained and preference established. The teacher's task is to offer the experience methodically in a sufficiently graded manner so that the discriminating ability of the pupils grows apace with (1) the reduced efforts of will and (2) the clear knowledge of self and ability to do that blow doubt and hesitation out of the way.

Go on trying to roll to the final position, applying the two means of checking and correcting yourself by projecting clearly (1) independence of the breath from the action as far as voluntary interference goes, and (2) the ability to reverse the motion of the body, bringing it back through the same trajectory continuously. From the beginning, all through the act, before and after it, the reversibility check should apply; that is, unstable equilibrium between excitation and inhibition should obtain at any instant. Perfection must not be expected or wished for. It is achieved by actually doing what is necessary to attain it, and by nothing else. It is impossible to perform an action involving the whole spine in absolute conformity to the two checks (breath and reversibility) without having achieved a highly coordinated use of self, and a working mastery of inhibiting unwanted contractions—which is the same as saying, without clearer motivation management. Time and experience are necessary for learning, and any shortcuts will compromise it. Only improving the method of teaching can reduce the time of apprenticeship.

While trying new modes of doing, until the one which is reversible is mastered, direct your attention to the sensations of the *body*. You will soon learn to distinguish quite clearly that lower abdominal fullness is necessary to make action possible without parasitic muscular tension in the whole body. The *acture* that feels easy, smooth, reversible, and spontaneously one's own is obtained when the point below the navel—roughly the center of gravity in the body—is sensed as the source or center of action. If this point is made the locus of the "I," in the sense we have explained, and the rest of the body is made subservient to allow for its displacement or its fixing in space, then coordinated, reversible, effortless motion will obtain in all action. The body feels weightless when the spine and the head are held without those contractions that are directly controlled by the will, contractions that shorten the spine for reasons other than the action itself.

It is hardly necessary to state that such concentrated learning as may be imagined from reading the preceding description would be enough to crush anybody. The whole procedure described lasts about ten minutes, the greatest part of which is passed in quiet attention and in a mood of playing about.

Now roll from the sitting position onto your back without making any other change in the relative position of the head, chest, or abdomen and without interference with your breath; that is, do not contract the abdomen to flatten it. If the movement is executed as described, your body tends to roll so as to bring the pelvis off the ground, and the body into balance on the shoulders and the head, provided the movement is slow. (Or you may completely roll over the head to bring your knees onto the ground. This full roll is rather rare, because most people contract the extensors of the back of the neck, and the head stops the body from rolling on.) Remain in each of the positions described at least for one minute, adjusting all the time your breath so that the movements are not interfered with by the chest becoming stiff.

16. Physiology and Social Order

Many things are so obvious that we rarely bother to think about their importance. The most apparently simple things are more complex than they seem, and their understanding makes life easier and more interesting. If a pound of potatoes costs a penny, two pounds cost twopence and ten pounds cost tenpence, that is simple enough. The scientist says, this is the law of proportionality. Well, the law of proportionality—perhaps the simplest law to understand—is in reality one of the most complex things when understood precisely. It works only if the amount of objects is so great that trading does not affect the total amount appreciably. The law of proportionality is applicable only to astronomical figures. When the number of free electrons available at any instant is small, as in a thin monomolecular line, Ohm's law (the current being proportionate to the applied voltage in a resistance) is not true any longer; the current fluctuates although the applied voltage is constant.

The complexity of the simple things is in reality so great that it would take a considerable amount of ingenuity and hard work to follow through the effects of the body's needing food and shelter on one's individual makeup. For we find an economic factor in every situation and in the most abstract thought, no matter how irrelevant the matter may seem at first sight. In the same way, the problem of sex affects almost every motive and deed. Adjustments to society, work, material and emotional security are closely linked with sexuality. Everybody knows about inferiority complexes. Little is necessary to convince anybody that inferiority or superiority feelings cannot arise without a society; one individual by himself is a norm unto himself. It is easy to conceive mentally that a feeling of inferiority may inhibit sexual potency. Impotence and frigidity can be, therefore, a social adjustment trouble and have no anatomical origin at all. Now, it is useful to know how sexual potency, which seems to be a purely physiological function, has anything to do with environment and social order. By knowing clearly what actually happens, we become better equipped to deal with failures of the mechanism.

When we are angry, frightened, fighting, bent on a task of importance, we are completely asexual. Wild animals often fight terrible battles before consummating the sexual act. Thus, after very strenuous physical efforts and often in a state of complete exhaustion, the sexual tension builds up, and the act is consummated. It is rather strange, to say the least of it, that it should happen this way.

Yet, in people the same thing happens. Historically, after bitter fighting, hunger, and deprivation, exhausted soldiers proceed to rape the women of conquered cities. Again, after periods of great tenseness and strain, there is an increase in sexual behavior. The increase in the number of births in wartimes is perhaps not unconnected with this thesis.

Striving, self-assertive financiers, theatrical artists, actors, and painters show greater sexuality than secretaries and civil servants. Even when the economic status of the former is precarious and inferior to that of the latter, they still manifest higher sexuality. When their efforts are particularly successful and they achieve public recognition, they are even more active than usual.

There is a common ground to all these seemingly unrelated things, namely a period of tense activity with heightened muscular tone, intense awareness of oneself, self-assertive integration, and self-protection, which is normally followed by an outburst of heightened sexuality. During the period of self-assertive activity, attention is directed to the action itself and any interference with it is resented; there is no room for any sexual thought or feeling. Such a state is obtained when the sympathetic nervous system is strongly excited. The body is fit for violent action through stimulation of this system, and the excitation of the system produces the necessary changes. The sympathetic system governs and tunes up the entire frame for finer protective and self-assertive action. Its stimulations increase the adrenalin content of the blood, accelerate the pulses, and increase muscular tone and awareness.

The parasympathetic system, as its name suggests, is intimately connected with the sympathetic in a reciprocal or antagonistic relationship; the stimulation of the first inhibits the second and *vice versa*. Many reactions in the body—the dilation of the pupils, for instance—can be produced in two ways: (1) by stimulating the sympathetic or (2) by inhibiting the parasympathetic, or inversely. The parasympathetic aids digestion, protects the eyes from excessive light, reduces muscular tone, slows down the heart, dilates the blood vessels, and, in general, controls the recuperative functions of the body. The two systems are in a seesaw relationship; the excitation balance shifts from one to the other, tuning up the entire frame now to strenuous efforts and then to restful recuperation.

This balance is largely influenced by our conscious attitude and action. When we speak of control of ourselves, we refer to our ability to influence one or the other of the systems to a more dominant state, fitting ourselves to the activity intended. The parasympathetic must be dominant and the sympathetic dormant before we can relax and become responsive to the opposite sex. As long as anything is stimulating the sympathetic system—that is, any agent that stimulates the protective and self-assertive functions vigorously enough—the sexual act is partially or completely inhibited.

All antagonistic or reciprocal functions show also the phenomenon of induction; that is, the longer one is excited, and consequently the other inhibited, the greater is the outburst of excitation once the inhibition is lifted. The time factor in induction is of primary importance. Thus, if we just glance at a black ink spot on a white sheet of paper, and then look at a clean white sheet, nothing in particular happens. But if we fix the black spot for about forty seconds or more, and then stare at the white sheet long enough (varying with different people from twenty to forty seconds), we perceive a white spot on the white paper, whiter than the paper. The time during which an action is maintained and the uniqueness of the action or its monochromatism, so to speak, are necessary to produce the phenomenon of induction. Extreme intensity nearing the threshold of pain also produces induction. In short, extreme or prolonged excitation confined to as monomotivated an action as possible gives rise to intense inhibition once the excitation is lifted. And, *vice versa,* prolonged and intense inhibition is followed by an outburst of excitation of the inhibited centers.

The two aspects of induction can be perceived in the preceding experiment. The black spot is surrounded by white; the first eliminates excitation, the other excites intensely. When we then look at the totally white surface, the spot becomes white and the surrounding area black. When either excitation or inhibition is maintained until fatigue sets in, the excited centers continue to be excited, and it is difficult to inhibit them; moreover, the inhibited centers continue to be inhibited, and it is difficult to excite them. The intervals of time and the intensities that produce induction or fatigue are essential properties of each individual nervous system, but like all other functional properties of the nervous system, they can be influenced by learning.

The two systems innervate most of the viscera, but not uniformly. The cervical and the sacral fibers that form the pelvic visceral nerves supply the large intestine, the rectum, and the bladder with motor fibers and the genitals with vasodilator fibers. These nerves and fibers constitute the parasympathetic system. Erection is caused by stimulation of the pelvic visceral nerves, which cause the dilation of the blood vessels of the penis and fill it with blood.

The experience suggested and the ones offered later on are designed to increase the range of control of the parasympathetic and to help the learner to recognize and control its dominance. The disentanglement of motivations is designed to sort them out into two groups: first, those motivations that belong to the dependence function associated with the protection and self-assertion of the individual, which are physiologically and habitually associated with sympathetic stimulation, and second, those that belong to the recuperative functions, which are restful and associated with poise and ease. The importance of monomotivation lies essentially in that the body-mind entity cannot at the same time be best fitted for both kinds of activity. In the neutral state, we are largely indifferent and are not motivated one way or the other. This state, and the means of shifting the balance at will, is what we are trying to learn to control.

The mental function is formed through the experience of the envelope of consciousness; thus the mental state and body state are functionally related, and the one reinstates the other as any part of a situation reinstates the whole. Both lines of approach must be equally used to obtain desired results.

The sexual act has two distinct functions: (1) reproduction and (2) regulation of the sympathetic-parasympathetic balance. This double function is rarely fully realized. It is usual to consider the sexual act as serving (1) the purpose of reproduction and (2) a lustful, pleasure-seeking urge that is legitimized or condoned in particular conditions. Powerful, self-assertive, and protective ability coincides with strong stimulation of the sympathetic, which when fatigued subsides and leaves the parasympathetic dominant. This reciprocity favors pronounced sexuality, power, possessiveness, greed, and lust. These qualities are indiscriminately lumped together and come to be considered as antisocial if not checked and moderated by society.

Pleasure or, more correctly, gratification accompanies and follows a proper sexual act, but there are more people than we can ever know to whom the sexual act invariably brings great disappointment, very little pleasure during the act, great moral frustration, and considerable physical discomfort. Yet they continue to inflict suffering on themselves. Certainly not for the sake of reproducing the human race, for everything possible is done to avoid pregnancy. They are urged to sexual activity not by the expectation of pleasure, which they rarely know, but by the need of relief and restfulness. The biological necessity for alternating first excitation and then rest of the two systems is sensed as an urge. And this balance is looked for whence it can come, so the normal and vigorous functioning of the two systems can be gained. For proper functioning, all nervous structure needs full activity followed by full rest. Such periodic swings are a general requirement for nervous activity, and we need only examine any function to confirm for ourselves that there is no exception to this rule.

Full gratification is the essence of the sexual act as far as the proper functioning of the system goes, for it comes only with sufficient stimulation of the parasympathetic. It has the same relationship to the act as taste does to food. The pleasure expectation is the urge to perform the biologically required act to maintain the orderly functioning of the system. Taste in food and sexual gratification are, from any other point of view, nonessential, but their absence interferes with feeding and normal nervous activity.

The protective functions and the recuperative ones make up an oscillating whole; the deeper the trough of the one, the higher the crest of the other. In normal everyday life in our society, the protective functions are exercised *not* in direct fighting, but in a drawn-out struggle and competition for economic independence or artistic recognition (which in the end means the same thing), as well as in other social activities. In all constructive human enterprise in a society such as ours, there is a competitive element that needs both organization of oneself and constant holding to a single idea and purpose, for which we can find no better expression than fighting. We fight "for peace," we have a Salvation Army, we fight "the battle of Christ," and we fight "our way to the top" of anything and to the foreground of everything. The expression seems to fit the attitude of those men and women who are bankers, industrialists, actors, painters, poets, and wrestlers. The attitude is the same as that of the fighting animal as far as the monochromatic stimulation and consequently the dominance of the sympathetic nervous system goes. And in the same way, we find increased sexuality in all driving, creative, single-minded people. Nothing can relieve and rest the sympathetic more than intense stimulation of the parasympathetic and the other way around. After a really good quarrel or fight, most couples find themselves sexually potent, and love is consummated more intensely than usual.

The intense stimulation of the parasympathetic produces orgasm; that is, involuntary contractions of the entire pelvic floor for both sexes, and in synchronism with male ejaculation of semen. The contractions of the pelvic floor are reflective, and any voluntary interference with the contractions of the anal sphincter, or with the involuntary movements of the pelvis itself, reduces and even stops the normal parasympathetic action. Orgasm, in such cases, is of lowered intensity or entirely absent and does not serve the biological purpose fully. The pleasurable sensation that is normally inseparable from orgasm thus dies before its time. The regulation of sympathetic-parasympathetic balance is disturbed, and instead of the normal response of intense gratification, which is normally attained when the parasympathetic builds up to the extreme and dies out in rhythmic steps, the sympathetic is brought into action by the self-assertive efforts of the will to succeed and the attempt to control oneself. Thus, instead of poise one feels irritation and disgust, muscular tension instead of relief.

The protective and self-assertive functions in a society such as ours are constantly overexcited during the dependence period to the point of becoming dominant motivations. During that period, the main recuperative reaction of the sexual act is inhibited in every way possible. The result is disturbance of the even shifting of dominance between the two groups of functions. Only when the protective and self-assertive functions are stimulated to the extreme, that is, to successful action in the field of social activity on which the person is bent, does the sympathetic system switch itself out sufficiently to allow the parasympathetic fuller stimulation, and fuller orgasm is obtained. Every person can recall in his own experience this sudden increase of potency that can be traced to particularly complete excitement of the protective and self-assertive functions. The muscular tenseness ceases, the breath becomes even, the lower abdomen feels full, and all the physiological symptoms of parasympathetic dominance follow, such as vasodilation and slow pulse. Irritation disappears, erection is more complete, and orgasm is more intense in the fuller quiescence of the sympathetic.

With this insight into the mechanism, we can understand how work, which often means little more than signing an occasional paper, and how, in general, interest in the world outside of ourselves have such a direct influence on our sexual behavior. Not only can we understand the connection between all the phenomena with which we began this chapter, but we can also see clearly the road to further improvements.

To get the right perspective of the situation, one must remember a cardinal physiological fact, namely fatigue of the nervous cells. If we concentrate intense activity on a small number of cells even for a short period, they fatigue. And the first degree of fatigue is not the refusal to function, but all-out activity. Thus, if we strain a small group of muscles by repeating exactly the same movement with the maximum intensity possible, the power falls off considerably after the sixth trial. However, the fatigue consists mainly in our inability to control the movement. The muscles do not become flabby and inactive, but on the contrary contract by themselves so often that they contract spasmodically, or cramp.

The same sort of thing happens in the first stage of fatigue of the cortical cells. If we think of one particular thing with great intensity for some time, the thought persists obsessively, and the cells continue to act once fatigued. Only by exciting another group of cells that will physiologically inhibit the fatigued ones, or after complete exhaustion, will the nagging thought cease. Pavlov's theory of the mosaic structure of the motor cortex of the brain provides a satisfactory explanation of these phenomena. In general, in order to produce any coordinated action some centers must be excited while the neighboring cells must be inhibited. The more definite and incisive the action, the smaller the number of cells that are active and the more complete the inhibition of the surrounding cells. A single cell completely excited fatigues rapidly, hence the difficulty of repeating, at will, perfect action with a single muscle in rapid succession.

When the self-assertive functions are continually overexcited, the sympathetic remains active and overstimulated by our efforts to relax. The fatigued cells continue to be excited and cannot be inhibited until they become completely exhausted. The overexcited brain loses the capacity for inhibition, hence sleeplessness and intense wishing to sleep make sleep impossible. This theory led Pavlov to devise his method of treating neurosis by induced and prolonged sleep.

We have here an explanation of the ill effects of overexciting the self-assertive function and the difficulty of recuperation we experience in such cases.

ON SEXUAL APPRENTICESHIP

Full orgasm accompanied by intense gratification is a physiological necessity for the smooth running of the protective, self-assertive, and recuperative functions. Physiologically, full orgasm is as important as procreation. From the standpoint of functioning of the individual frame, it even takes precedence over procreation, for parenthood in conditions of improper adjustment to society is a handicap both to the parents and the offspring. A smooth balance between the self-assertive and recuperative functions cannot be obtained in persons without the ability of full orgasm. Without full orgasm, there is no biological function fulfilled; such sexual intercourse does nothing but lower the vitality of the entire frame. No matter how varied one's life may otherwise be, without the occasional absolute abandonment of the protective and self-assertive habits—as occurs only in frank, spontaneous, and harmonious relationship between a man and a woman—there always remains an anxious longing for something sensed as an ideal state of peaceful well-being.

In most cases of impotence and frigidity, we find—in the final analysis—an improper social integration. Female and male friendships in these cases are superficial and circumstantial; the person is too self-centered and at the same time terribly greedy for affection. The internal conflict between self-assertion and sociability has never been emotionally solved other than through suppression of now one, now the other, of the impulses. Social integration and sexuality are essentially the same thing. The sexual function is the biological expression of the drive for intercourse and communion with other individuals. The most extreme individualist must forgo some self-sufficiency to make sexual relationship possible. Proper social integration requires an awareness that our personal well-being depends on others.

The problem is, of course, a many-sided one; civilizations are the different modes of solving it. None of the solutions has enjoyed undivided success; all have had difficulties. But those persisting have considerable advantages that secure and sustain their existence. In our own civilization sexual maturity does not seal the period of economic dependence on parents, so that the physiologically adult person lingers on for a considerable period in infantile dependence. Social integration and sex are therefore intimately linked in all of us, on that account alone, although in reality this is only one of many links.

In our education, self-assertion is taught as an unadulterated benediction, yet sex and economics remain mutually exclusive during the formation of the sexual function. During this period, instead of the guidance one is in most need of, one is taught inhibition of self. Conflict is sown continuously by everyone who can lend a hand to it, and the tradition is not to hand on tradition, forcing everyone to start from the beginning in the most unfavorable conditions.

Thus, the sexually mature adolescent is compelled to emphasize self-assertiveness in order to obtain social condonation of sexual aspirations. In most cases of trouble in the sexual function, an essential problem in social adjustment is usually found, which may be outwardly perfect, but is nevertheless emotionally unsatisfactory. It is necessary to further the social standing and the economic independence of such persons, as the active cultivation of proper self-assertiveness leads to a direct improvement in the sexual trouble. The higher the level of social integration (no matter, of course, what the occupation is), the higher will be the sexual tension consequently built up.

It is an absolute necessity, therefore, for everyone to learn to distinguish compulsive self-assertive motivations that are carried on and actively maintained when they should, in fact, be given up so that parasympathetic dominance may be allowed full freedom.

We have now before us a clear program. Faltering erection, lukewarm orgasm, frigidity and lifelessness will not be sustained when the freedom of sympathetic and parasympathetic flow is established. Proper self-assertiveness must be actively cultivated, and learning and exercising of this function is the only actual improvement. We must and can learn to feel and control parasympathetic dominance in order to learn to distinguish those self-assertive and protective motivations that excite the sympathetic and hinder erection and full orgasm. We must also learn to distinguish the unrecognized habitual motivations of self-assertion sustaining muscular tensions that interfere directly with the involuntary contractions of the pelvic floor, lower abdomen, hips, and anal sphincter and never allow orgasm to build. In short, we must learn an orderly and smooth control of our entire frame, emotions, and muscles that are one and the same functional whole.

It must be understood that it is not the actual contraction of the muscles that is the interfering agent, but (1) the constantly excited points of the cortex and (2) the permanently inhibited ones, that interfere with the free flow of excitation and inhibition and make monomotivated functioning impossible. Every new pattern that we project has first to comply with these and be compromised (so as to allow the unrecognized habitual points of rigidity to remain undisturbed) before we can enact it. The result is that sensation of being tied down and unable to change that is expressed so vividly in that popular saying, "The more we change, the more we stay the same."

Muscular control is the thing in which we have the greatest experience. The result of a new attitude is at once sensed in the personal language of the individual. The influence on the vegetative state is very direct as the pulse, breathing, and vascular state are involved at once and at the same time. It is easier to disentangle motivation crossings once the feel of them is recognized by the person in his own body, than by verbal analysis where we have to look for symbolism to help us to understand what the person really feels and means by what he says. The new action must first be experienced in conditions such that the person recognizes comfort in the new action and discomfort in the habitual one. An important advantage in beginning with muscular control of the body is that in this domain we can quite convincingly *show* what the correct action is, without arousing opposition.

We have the choice of two methods of approach: pick on the most flagrant faults and correct them one by one, or proceed systematically. When all the advantages of either of these methods are weighed, the second of the two is always to be preferred. We have been following this line of thought up to now.

The first thing to do is to restore to the pelvis full mobility. The pelvis supports the whole weight of the body, and in that respect is the most important part of it. The head, in which all of the most precise organs of orientation are located, cannot be properly held without the pelvis supporting the body so that no unnecessary muscular strain exists all along the spine. Without proper pelvic control, adjustment of the head carriage is a laborious and thankless job. Control of the head is indispensable for the finest use of the self; we in fact started with lifting the head off the ground. But already in this simple movement one must first anchor the chest to the pelvis before the head can be lifted. It is rather futile to bring in the question of priority, for the contractions are practically simultaneous, although strictly speaking, the pelvic muscles are the first to contract in all extensive and rapid movements and the head moves first in slow ones.

By establishing the full range of mobility and control of the pelvic region, we lift fixity of state from the cortical centers and facilitate thereby the realization of the projected acts; thus, reversibility of the entire frame is improved. Men and women capable of full orgasm have a better control of the pelvis than others. Their gait and movements in general are less strained, their *acture* simpler and easier. On the other hand, people suffering from any sexual difficulties have the pelvis more or less immobile, and some patterns of its movement are completely inhibited. Some people have the movement corresponding to forward coitus or full penetration practically excluded from normal use, to the extent of permanently holding the pelvis in the position of withdrawal. Others hold the pelvis continuously in the position of complete penetration with the hip joints completely extended. In both cases the motivation for normal intercourse is distorted or absent. The person does not act spontaneously, but for all sorts of extraneous reasons belonging to the domain of self-assertion. The action is not dictated nor maintained by gratification. In the first case, the motivation for coitus is crossed with that of self-deprecation or weakness, guilt or shame, or conviction of ugliness. Both persons have great difficulty in showing themselves nude to the partner, especially the male when he is not in a state of full erection. When naked, they both tense and lose what little spontaneity they are normally capable of through correct adjustment. In the second case, the person is so anxious for coitus, doubting that it will last long enough or ever happen again, that penetration is demanded as soon as the erection is more or less complete. Such persons are miserable, as the woman experiences only lifelessness in the pelvic region, and the man ejaculates immediately after penetration in accordance with the dominant motivation present at the moment. They project the idea of orgasm as the essence of the act, whereas, in proper *acture,* the onset of orgasm is of no more conscious concern to the person than swallowing saliva at that moment. The rhythmic movements of forward coitus, or penetration and withdrawal, are not even contemplated in improper *acture:* the person is either motionless or in violent, jerky agitation, with the body stiffened in the habitual muscular pattern. Rhythmic movements are impossible in any action whatsoever so long as the pelvis is maintained rigidly. The vicious circle of the actual body sustaining the mental and vegetative state that it reflects holds the person under strain and feeling dominated by an evil power.

The importance of freeing the pelvis from habitual contractions thus becomes obvious. It is not because of any intrinsic quality of this or that position of the pelvis. Once compulsiveness is lifted, any contraction is compatible with normal functioning, and any contraction, however awkward, is only a minor discomfort. The freeing is necessary in order to lift the habitual compulsive pattern in the attitude of the person to the act. That attitude is dissolved with the dissolution of the cortical pattern formed through the exclusion of the mobility of the pelvis. Because as long as this immobility persists, the person, not recognizing the mental state, is unaware of what reinstates the failure this time—as if a devil had been at the works and spoiled them internally without any visible sign of his malice, so that failure appears only in actual use. Without direct muscular readjustment, it is a question of trial and error. The dissolution of emotional complexes slowly resolves anxiety, and the muscular tension disappears; that is, the constantly excited cortical centers begin to function normally—and action finally becomes smoother and easier. In this case the person may become aware of the existence of the tension and remove it, yet not realize what is actually happening. A period of success and failure follows therefore and every failure brings the person back to ground zero. Learning to recognize what is actually happening and gaining direct control over it makes success and failure into acts, as opposed to happenings.

Without this awareness, every relapse brings the person back into psychiatric treatment, for shorter periods of time—at least until the next relapse. With any sort of skillful treatment, the anxiety of failure is eventually reduced, and relapses become less intense. By and by the desired state is reached at the expense of great misery, which could be avoided by a more direct learning.

CLARIFYING SOME NOTIONS

In all human functions that need apprenticeship, such as love, hatred, speaking, thinking, walking, sitting, sex, and others, no part of that apprenticeship can be skipped with complete impunity. Sometimes, of course, with special luck and in habitual unchanging conditions, one may get away with it. Normally, however, in the fumbling with and exploring of the full range of each function, making mistakes is essential to satisfactory learning. During the apprenticeship, mistakes are correct action; they are agreed on and are part of the business. One cannot become a past master of any field of human endeavor without the most important item of learning how to do, which is the personal experience of what *not* to do. The teacher's job is only to preserve the pupil from fatal mistakes or those which will cause permanent injury.

In many cases of inability to do, an essential part of personal experience is lacking. The person is compelled to follow very closely a procedure that must not be deviated from, even in the minutest detail. Such action is to all intents and purposes compulsive in character, and the person is continually running the danger of failure. Sexual behavior for most of us suffers from this sort of fault. It cannot be corrected permanently and satisfactorily without working through the skipped part of normal apprenticeship.

In most cases, however, young people have an appreciable apprenticeship in courtship, dancing, kissing, and petting with more or less intimate contact. Thus the final step is not such an entirely new and trying task.

Most people suffering from sexual incompetence belong, on the one hand, to the group of those who have braved society too early and, on the other hand, to those who have been more Catholic than the pope, and have not taken advantage of, but have, in fact, skipped the permissible bridging courtship apprenticeship. Sexually incompetent people have this in common—the development of the sexual function was not evenly spread in time, and they faced a task that was (and still is) much above their head.

Their position is similar to that of the self-educated person. In some ways such persons are much above their fellow men who had a normal and formal schooling. And occasionally they pull it off and become the fairy-tale self-made men and women. But the number of wrecks having this self-miseducation, who lead miserable lives, feeling that they could reach great heights if only they were recognized, is considerable. Their trouble is not lack of recognition, but the lack of skill that one comes by only through proper apprenticeship. Very capable men or women often ruin their lives just by skipping or passing too rapidly through some part of the normal apprenticeship. I know some extremely gifted engineers who cannot reach the position they deserve, just because they have been foolish enough to think that it is enough to understand mechanics and mathematics and have therefore totally neglected the drudgery of working out examples. They still have their mechanical ingenuity, but all they can do is make inventions without being able to bring them to a successful final marketable product. The sooner they sit down to close the gap in their apprenticeship, the better is their chance of getting what is rightfully within their reach.

Take, for example, the case of the man who never helps bring his wife to feel full orgasm. He may be advised by his doctor, or may have found in a book, that women need to be caressed, kissed, and cuddled before the act. The fact that he does not do these things, which are supposed to come "naturally," shows that he has never felt the confidence or the ability to do so. He is put to the test, and so he approaches his partner in a mood that has nothing in common with that of a mature male in the same position. He proceeds now to follow instructions that he got, most probably without any spontaneous desire to do so, and before long he returns to his habitual procedure with the habitual result.

In all learned acts that do not bring the desired result, an essential part of the apprenticeship has been skipped and only understood intellectually, instead of having been worked through. The sooner that is remedied, the better.

In most acts we can see other people's efforts, their errors, the way they correct them. There are teachers and pupils. In the sexual act, this is impossible; the social pattern is such that if somebody attempted to open a practical school its usefulness would be very doubtful, even if there were no public censure and it were allowed to function. The teaching would necessarily take a form that has little to do with traditional procedure, so that the learned procedure could rarely be used in normal conditions. Unless both man and woman were students of the same school, the procedure would be more of a handicap than a help. Such a couple would be so entirely dependent on each other that their antagonism and resentment would certainly grow in both of them until only discord existed between them. Moreover, they would feel different from everybody else and, therefore, abnormal. The more one contemplates the possibility, the more one finds objections to it; hence the nonexistence of such institutions.

Before finding a way out, let us see briefly what the normal apprenticeship consists of. In early childhood, both males and females become aware of their sexual organs and manipulate them. These manipulations have little origin other than the greater sensitivity of these parts and the special sensation they produce. This manipulation is the normal course of sexual apprenticeship, as much as crawling is the normal way of learning to walk. As Malinowski has shown to be the case in some tribes, the next step is the manipulation of the erogenous zones of the opposite sex. Many people never further their sexual function beyond self-masturbation. Even more people stop their development at the petting stage and are completely satisfied when they bring the partner to orgasm mainly through caressing and kissing. In primitive societies, there is a gradual passing from manipulation to penetration, which is at first faltering. Only slowly does the full erective potency replace the earlier forms of sexual gratification. By and by, unobtrusively and without any more sense of failure or success than in learning walking, the person arrives at the final stage of apprenticeship in which sexual gratification culminates in full orgasm of both partners with that friendliness and mutual feeling of intimacy that always results from the complete abandonment of self-assertiveness; where virile pride and feminine passivity are thrown overboard without any attempt to do so.

In our society sexual apprenticeship is barred until the final crucial test. The first intercourse takes place when the person considers himself and is considered by others to be an adult. He is expected to have an innate "instinct" that will do everything for him in a way "that comes naturally," whereas, in fact, he has only an urge that comes naturally. And even the form that the urge takes in every individual is so influenced by personal history that the word *natural* in this context is more a manner of speech than a description of a fact.

Some individuals do dare to infringe on the social prohibition of sexual intercourse in early childhood. But they are not much better off than the others, for a series of extraneous emotional stresses become associated with sexual activity. If they are female, they must steal their gratification and their partner loses the respect for them that he has for other women. They often feel guilty and find themselves incapable of obtaining the same gratification in socially more acceptable conditions.

In readjusting the sexual function to normal maturity without going through the intermediary stages, one is up against the same difficulty as in trying to become a perfect tennis player straight away without first having gone through the clumsy and faulty movements that must be discarded before the correct movements can be preferred by the body sensations as something better. Or as if one were to try to design a perfect chair without ever having sat on chairs before. My contention is that in all cases of normal sexual behavior this course of apprenticeship has been gone through at least more or less haphazardly, or else it takes place in the early stages of marriage. Many failures of any real improvement in cases of frigidity and impotence are due to the neglect of this essential learning, and no amount of analysis will bring about any improvement in functioning if it does not bring the person through a shortened course of such apprenticeship.

In all cases where the apprenticeship has been scanty, hurried, or even skipped, the sexual problem is central for the person. It always involves sufficient mobilization of self-assertion to make full orgasm rare or even impossible. In healthy development, the sexual problem is simple (leaving the central position which it occupies almost entirely in other cases), so that the person can direct his whole being and energy in an evolving manner, growing in power and experience. At times, after the self-assertive state of *acture* has been fully and wholeheartedly (and therefore successfully) enjoyed, the sexual activity per se does not occupy a central position, but the entire being is completely abandoned in unreserved intimacy, which is the only way in which orgasm can produce the harmonious functioning of the entire nervous system. Once this is achieved there is no tension, and the whole problem is relegated to its proper place to remain dormant in the shadow of consciousness.

In correct behavior, sexual activity is as essential as blood circulation. Likewise, it does not push itself to the foreground ("the wave") of our awareness unless there is trouble. From the beginning of learning how to better use the self, one should employ the released vitality for good purpose, as this directly improves *acture* which in turn, increases vitality. The most important use one can make of this released energy is to increase one's security, *economic* and *emotional* as they amount to the same thing. This means not simply work, but making oneself irreplaceable at it. If there is a problem, and therefore one's occupation is not congenial, it must be changed—but only after one has been through whatever anonymous motivations are at the back of both troubles. This may be difficult to do, and it should therefore be left until the general state has improved and the emotional difficulty solved. The necessary steps to be taken will then become self-evident. In every profession there is room for creative self-application, even in doing nothing, provided the occupation suits one. It is easier to give this advice than to abide by it. And everybody has probably been through this sort of thing before, but when reasoning is clouded by cross motivations, all solutions are found equally attractive one second, and equally objectionable or completely uninteresting the next. The dissolution of any unrecognized motivation, if it results in some change you make in your environment—even a change no more drastic than the way of eating, breathing, diet, or sleeping— is a good omen for a better future. A man, like any living thing, can thrive only in a medium with fitting conditions, and mature men change their environment to suit themselves and are flexible in body and spirit in order to be able to cope with a wide variety of conditions. Poise or improvement cannot increase, nor even persist for very long, unless one alters the environment so that the old habitual response is not reinstated. If the old habit is sustained by the environment, it will persist like a corn on the foot which grows again so long as there is pressure, making the corn a sign of healthy and correct adjustment to an unhealthy and painful condition.

If a person finds nothing to interest him deeply, there is little doubt that conflicting motivations are at work—there is no dominant one, so no action can be taken, and no interest can arise. Currently there is a trend toward achieving things through intellectual effort and skipping apprenticeship on all levels of activity in general and sexual activity in particular. But it is no use making will efforts; they solve nothing. The correct approach is to disentangle at least one thread of the knot of cross motivation, and then at once one discovers more hidden treasures of capacity and vitality in oneself than anybody suspected. Our society would not exist if there were not room for every person, no matter who he is, to live fully. For example, self-critical people, who do not find room for themselves (and unbeknownst to them, do not believe in themselves), believe that the world is made for them, that they are unique, unrecognized, and better than anybody else they know. Paradoxically (at first sight), people who find fault with themselves also find themselves to be better than anybody else.

The world is quite interesting when you learn to influence it ever so little. There is so much to do to make this world fit for ourselves that we cannot afford to have thinking people wasting themselves away in sterile internal struggles. Obviously, something must be done about changing and improving education and the social order that dictates it so that the havoc wreaked in many minds is not perpetuated. But to make this change possible the present generation must do something to itself to become free from those beliefs that sustain misery and impotence. In most cases of impotence and frigidity in all their forms (except in a few cases of congenital anatomical deformation), the sufferers are the victims of improper teaching and incorrect learning. This has necessitated a deformation of personality in demanding from it more than it could give without providing the means for complying with these demands. Understanding this should lift enough anxiety to enable most people to set about learning the right manner of *acture.* But to achieve maturity one must be prepared to change and give up cherished beliefs and habits (these old patterns may be taken up again later once their compulsiveness is lifted).

People often fail to derive all the benefits of any method of readjustment, because they want to both change themselves and at the same time remain as they are. This is not only the result of believing that they can keep their habitual personality and change only those features of their behavior that they do not like (whereas in fact a radical change of acture always entails a change of mental attitude, the way of projecting action, voice, breathing, and muscular effort), but it is also the result of habitual inertia. One always can produce a sufficient explanation to oneself for confirming the rationality of one's own behavior in all the daily acts. Only by learning to recognize and disentangle motivations through experiencing their effect on the body state and *acture* can one get rid of compulsion and habitual, machinelike subservience to habit.

People who refuse to consider the tendency to change and force themselves to the habitual rationalization of their *acture* in the small daily acts nip in the bud any transfer of learning. The transfer of learning is especially important in sexual apprenticeship, which cannot be taught by actual practice without creating new and great difficulties. The learner is always left to be his own judge at the very moment when objective judgment would be most valuable. There is no other way to correct faulty *acture* in general than by weeding out compulsiveness through learning reversibility.

Reversibility is obtained when the reciprocal functions of excitation and inhibition are in a state of unstable equilibrium, from which volitional control is easy. Near the state of equilibrium, little effort is necessary to shift the balance in any direction, because unstable balance corresponds to the configuration where a system has its maximal potential energy. All we have learned earlier is now useful for this purpose. The facts that (1) the mental functions are formed through the individual experience of the frame, so that cerebral functioning corresponds to body states, and that (2) the conscious control enables us to dissociate the cerebral functioning from the executive frame or allow the reinstatement of the situation as it occurred (or any other configuration we choose), give us a powerful and convenient means of learning through mental activity, while the enaction of the cortical impulses by the musculature is inhibited. (In this conjunction, let the reader recall the example of learning to play the piano without striking the keys.)

This inhibition of physical action while formulating the projected action is one of the most effective means of correct learning used by all normal and skillful people. *An act performed escapes at once into the past, where it becomes completely immune and beyond reach.* We can compensate for or correct the effect of a past act by a new act, but we can never bring back the first act and correct it. All skilled people having good *acture* have learned to manage their motivation capital before allowing action to take place. And it is necessary to learn this dissociation of direction of oneself from enacting the directions until the dissociation becomes so familiar and rapid as to be practically simultaneous with the action. At that stage, our action is spontaneous without internal resistance and without parasitic motivations.

When learning a new pattern of *acture*, it is necessary to bring oneself nearer to the *acture* of reversibility, even in the act of learning. At the moment of acting, one must learn to reject the furthering of the action; reversibility is thus roughly attained, just enough to remove the intense compulsiveness. At this moment we can become aware of the flagrant muscular tension and the motivation behind it. The muscular tension can now be inhibited, and the frame can be brought nearer to the tonic state of *acture.* Reduced tension entails higher suggestibility; that is, easier direction or control in nonassertive direction of self, which means that reversibility has further improved. From previous learning we know that these states correspond to parasympathetic dominance, which is thus being brought about.

Thus, each state leads the frame onto the other. From the point of view of inhibition and excitation, the state of the cortex facilitates the elimination of tension, and the reduction of tension brings about a more reversible state. Tension is further reduced, and breath becomes rhythmical; in short, the whole frame is geared up in such a way as to tune it for easy smooth control. The projection is poised, the body is held in tonic *acture,* the body is warm, the forehead is cool, there is no awareness of any discrete part of self, the entire being feels a single whole, the lower abdomen feels to be the source of self, with the pelvis leading in all motion—and thus spontaneous *acture* is achieved.

THE VICIOUS CIRCLE

In the whole discussion up till now, there has been no mention of the fact that sexual relations are not the private affair of one individual, but an experience involving a partner of the opposite sex. That partner grows in similar conditions of dependence, and therefore we find that corresponding modes of behavior are cultivated. The two sets of behavior must sustain each other in order to exist. Sexual incompetence in one is fostered by the respective reaction of the partner, which makes the incorrect response a necessary one.

The woman's need for help and protection during pregnancy and after giving birth to her child fosters such a mode of behavior that it sustains in the male a motivation to act to that effect. The habitual dependence patterns—which are parasitic as far as the purely sexual motivation is concerned, and which must be cast away to attain correct action—are thus reinstated by the partner's needs, whether she is aware of it or not.

The purity of sexual motivation is, therefore, extremely difficult to maintain in the present form of male-female dependence relationship in our society. Sexual incompetence is sustained by this vicious circle.

It is instructive to follow the different modes and patterns of dependence in our society. The body tension that needs the sexual act in order to be released is quite catholic and imposes only one condition on the partner, namely sufficient sexual competence to release the tension adequately. The more fundamental condition of assisting the internal building up of body tension or excitation to an intensity sufficient to produce the involuntary reflective contraction of orgasm, is self understood, though often neglected. Without the body tension, there is no room for body tension release. Many people struggle futilely, trying to build up sexual body tension by an internal effort of "will" or imagination, whereas it should and can be achieved only by the environment's sustaining the proper response, that is, by the partner's being equally brought to act by an unswamped sexual motivation.

In practice, however, the habitual dependence pattern restricts the choice of a partner to extremely narrow limits. The economic status of the partner, the race, religion, nationality, social standing, fashion, and all sorts of other habitual patterns restrict the choice to such narrow limits that only the competent mature adult actually chooses a partner. The great majority of people have the choice made for them by motivations that contradict the sexual one. The incompetent person has the sexual motivations so deeply buried under the parasitic ones that the choice is often limited to an imaginary partner who is not to be found anywhere. The strictness of choice to which the person is addicted is the measure of that person's incompetence.

Thus, the incompetent person finds it impossible to decide (with so many contradictory motivations continually at work) who is the partner that is really wanted. The sexual motivation makes most partners acceptable, while the contradictory motivations reject most of them. This vicious circle is sustained, with the incompetent person enacting all the contradictory motivations perpetuating incompetence.

17. The Abdomen, the Pelvis, and the Head

The spine is carried by the pelvis. The head rides like a plate at the upper end of a Chinese juggler's bamboo rod. All that constitutes the body hangs from the spine or from the ribs, which themselves hang from the spine. The pelvis is, therefore, the carrier of the lot. No proper action is possible without good control of the pelvic joints. The strongest muscles of the body articulate the pelvic joints; the gluteals (or buttock muscles) and the quadriceps (or big thigh muscles) have the largest cross sections of all the muscles. In short, the power of a body is determined by the power of the lower abdomen and more generally by the pelvic region. In correct action, the work done is distributed so that the big muscles do a bigger share of the work and the smaller ones do less in proportion to their size. All action that feels easy and does not produce the sensation of muscle strain is so performed. All action that feels strenuous calls on the smaller muscles of the periphery of the body, such as the hands, feet, arms, and legs, to do a greater share of the work than they should. The *acture* is then such that the pelvis is fixed in some way or other and is not allowed to carry the weight of the spine longitudinally, as it should.

No correct posture or *acture* is possible without the pelvis being able to move freely in all its articulations; that is, in the hip joints and in the small of the back. As soon as one of the possible motions of the pelvis is restrained, the fluency of action is broken. Thereafter, great efforts in the shoulder girdle or in the legs are necessary to accomplish what can be done with grace and ease when pelvic mobility is unhampered. Moreover, no exertion can replace correct pelvic motion as far as the quality of action is concerned. Some great judo experts are past masters in the art of pelvic control, and the ascendancy they have over less skillful people is bewildering.

There is perhaps no other part of the body about which so many half-truths have been and are being said as the abdomen. For some schools, it has to be as flat and as taut as a board; drawing it in is almost universally recommended. Here again, I think judo masters are nearer to the correct understanding of its functioning than any other school, and some of them have an ideal control of it. The heavy contents of the abdominal area, the lungs, the heart and vocal apparatus, are all hanging from the spine in the last resort, as are all the muscles that hold them. The abdominal content proper, which is everything below the diaphragm, is also supported by the pelvic floor muscles. All these muscles must be tonically contracted; that is, their degree of tension should not be interfered with by voluntary action. If the spine and head are held properly, the tension in the pelvic floor, abdomen, diaphragm, throat, and tongue is determined by their weight, and any interference by voluntary drawing in, stiffening, or pushing forward is incompatible with correct posture. Such alterations of the muscular tone of the abdominal region are only necessary for particular purposes. In standing or sitting, nothing should be done with any part of the body except standing or sitting. The conscious control should be used to eliminate all parasitic contraction that may linger on from habits inculcated by imitating or complying with dogmatic and rigid people.

The taut abdomen school refers to the flat abdomen of ancient Greek sculpture as a prototype of perfection. Most Greek statues do in fact show very good *acture* (in the case of statues, *posture* would probably be equally correct), but you will notice by careful examination that their abdomens are held free from voluntary tightening. The lower abdomen is full; that is, one can sense the viscera resting against the abdomen and weighing on the abdominal wall. The muscles are drawn up by this weight tonically. To produce the same degree of abdominal flatness by voluntary contraction (by pulling the abdomen in or up) either the pelvis is tilted with its top too far back, or the chest is made rigid and the lower ribs protrude too far forward.

In fact, it is quite futile to talk of correctly holding the abdomen, the pelvis, the chest, or the neck *individually.* So long as there is holding in any one of them, all the others are being held to some degree so that whatever act is undertaken it must be performed in spite of this holding, and is therefore poorly coordinated.

The head rides on the top of the spine. It is maintained in its position by the neck muscles, the weight of the head automatically dictating the right tone to maintain it so that the vestibular apparatus in the ear can detect both the slightest deviation from the vertical and any minute changes in uniformity of motion; that is, changes of velocity and acceleration. When the head is correctly correlated with the body, there is no contraction that can be reduced directly by volition without directing a change of position of the head. The head floats freely with the smoothness of a cork floating on water. The mechanical importance of the head in *acture* is capital.

The head carries all the double-organ sense apparatus which connect us with the distant world, and which are therefore referred to as *teleceptors.* Information from the outside world is useless if we do not know immediately the direction from which it is issued and its distance. Two organs separated from each other are necessary for stereoscopic vision and the appreciation of direction and distance of sound. Both the eyes and the ears are so innervated that the head turns reflectively until the two organs in each case are equally excited by the signal coming from the distant disturbance. The eyes, in particular, move together so that the images of the focused object formed on the retinas overlap always in the same manner.

The head is capable of following the eyes without delay, in spite of its inertia and weight, as it is articulated near its centers of gravity and inertia. And the excitation of the eyes or the ears increases the tone of the neck muscles so that the head can be turned at the expense of its potential energy (except when looking straight up) with the muscles only directing the "fall" of the head most of the time.

The eyes have an overriding control over the neck reflexes. Overriding controls are generally more delicate and permit finer gradation of movement when time allows their use. If you make as little effort as possible so that you can begin to distinguish finer shades of sensations, you may be able to detect a considerable difference between the following two movements. First, move your head together with your eyes to the right. Repeat a few times, and notice the sharp clicking motion of the head as if it were moving between two stops. Second, move your head to the right, but this time use your eyes to scan the horizon uninterruptedly as swiftly as you like before fixing them in the direction in which the head stopped in the previous experiment. You will notice, by alternately repeating the two movements, that when the eyes are used the head moves smoothly all through the movement. Also, you can reverse the movement of the head at any point without effort when the eyes are used for looking first and the head turns to follow them. On the other hand, there is real difficulty in reversing the movement of the head before it comes to the right stop, if you are not leading with the eyes, unless you decide so beforehand.

These simple experiments show quite clearly two distinguishing features of the human nervous system: namely, (1) the overriding influence of the eye reflexes over the neck reflexes and (2) the still higher overriding influence of conscious volition that enables us to release eye control and leave the lower neck reflexes to manage it their own way (or to interrupt this momentary appointment to mastership and put the eyes at the helm when we wish). When the incoming signal is unexpected or of exceptional violence, the neck reflexes act automatically. In normal awareness, the eyes are the leaders. In the higher animals, such as apes, the eyes play a role similar to that in men. In lower animals, such as rabbits, the neck reflexes play a much more autonomous role, and the position of the head on the body determines the tone in the rest of the body.

General features of proper use of the self can now be formulated. The head should remain absolutely free to float riding on the top of the spine. All tension in the neck and the throat interferes with the motion of the head and makes coordinated action more or less imperfect. The atlas—the top of the spine—should always point in the direction of the point on the top of the skull where a water jet coming up through the spine would hit the skull when the head is being balanced in the standing position without voluntary tension anywhere in the body from the pelvis upward. Later we shall give some indications by which to identify the sensation corresponding to the proper alignment.

The most frequent cause for tension in the neck is the fear of failure; that is, such tension expresses an intimate realization of the inability to act adequately. The person mobilizes all his power and acts too quickly and too intently, believing that this will assure success. Such action lacks gradation and coordination; hurry and effort are no substitute for skill. They always indicate the presence of doubt of one's own ability to cope with the situation. The motivation to succeed is, in such cases, stronger than the motivation to act. Failure is the necessary corollary of correct action; without it, correct action has no meaning. Failure is eliminated by correct action, not by fear of failure. In correct *acture,* the alternative of failure has no compulsive tension about it. When the fear of failure is an emotive constituent of all action, as a compulsive habitual attitude can be, personal security is hinged on it. The person is so critical and biased against himself that he often sees failure where objective observers fail to detect it. The person feels the internal tension just described and is aware of something being wrong, although he cannot identify the problem in terms of muscular tension that is depressing the head or another spinal joint. When he learns to recognize the parasitic action and the origin of its compulsive presence, he regains conscious control over it, and spontaneity is restored.

ABDOMINAL CONTROL

It is very difficult to convey a precise idea of proper abdominal control without personal contact. The only way to do so is to invite the reader to do certain acts or adopt certain attitudes, and to rely on his ability to feel the difference between these various states of his own body, and to finally discover for himself what is meant.

The external visible or tangible differences are too small to be detected except by the trained teacher.

It is very important to realize that there is no mystery here, or secret control unknown to common mortals except "experts." An expert can only use methodically what everyone else does by chance every now and then. But chance fails in use when wished for, because unlike the expert, most people do not know exactly what they are doing, and therefore they cannot learn to control it. We all have occasional spells when we feel ease, grace, and power at the same time; we are in "good form." At that moment our control is better than usual, and we are capable of a more satisfactory use of ourselves. We want to be able to reproduce such states at will, as some people do, without any difficulty at all. Such people are rare, and we are inclined to think that they have something we don't have, when in reality the only difference is that they can regularly use and maintain a manner of self-direction that we have only now and then for short spells. Now obviously we cannot learn the use of something that we do not have at all.

Abdominal control, then, begins thus. When you are swinging an axe overhead with both hands, just at the moment when the axe changes direction and begins to move on its downward path, your abdomen is in the right state of contraction. This holds true only provided that the arms are not consciously contracted and the chest is held so that the swing forward expels air freely from the lungs. Try the movement without an axe a number of times, and then stop at the instant described, with both hands above the head. Observe the state of contraction of the lower abdomen. The position of the pelvis and the state of the lower abdomen are as near as possible to what we have in mind.

Sit on a chair with your feet apart, the thighs at right angles to each other. Look straight ahead. Then put your hands on your knees and slump your back until it touches the back of the chair in the lumbar region. Push your lower abdomen forward by a sudden contraction so that air is expelled freely from your lungs through the mouth, somewhat in the manner of the bark or cough of a dog. Carefully observe yourself and you will notice that your shoulders

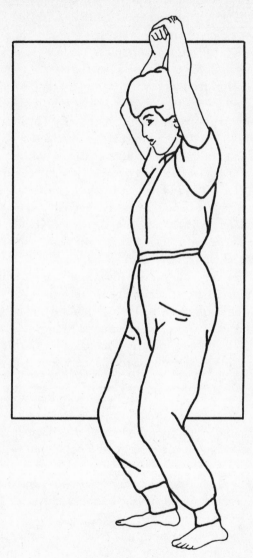

When swinging an axe overhead with both hands (just at the moment when the axe changes direction and begins to move on its downward path).

stiffen, the back of the head pulls toward the nape, and the chin protrudes well in front of your abdomen. Repeat this several times. Then push your lower abdomen sharply forward once more, expelling air freely, and remain motionless for a few seconds, observing and taking notice of the fullness and the state of contraction of the abdomen. Now remove your back from the chair back, bringing your lower abdomen further forward still. Your back arches, and another puff of air is expelled from your lungs. The head is raised and brought into vertical alignment, the shoulders relax, and the tense contraction of the lower abdomen ceases but it remains full and rounded. If your breath has become easy and rhythmic, your shoulders are lying still and feel loose, and your head is capable of following your eyes to about forty-five degrees behind your right and left shoulders without any change whatsoever of your neck, shoulders, and chin, you have got it right again.

Repeat the whole procedure several times. The test of correctness consists in that you can remain in the final attitude for two or three minutes without sensing strain or feeling a tendency to correct yourself. Moreover, while maintaining this attitude your face muscles should relax and a sense of poise should pervade you. The sense of well-being becomes more and more pronounced while waiting. If time seems long to you, then start it all over again —you have not got it.

Now lean your back against the chair, again slouching your head forward with the lumbar vertebrae resting against the back of the chair. Put your hands on your thighs near the abdomen; close your eyes. It is essential that the chair should not be too high for you; that is, the hamstrings of your thighs should not be compressed by the weight of the thighs. If necessary, put something under your feet so that you sit only on the buttocks and not on the thighs at the same time.

Close your mouth, the teeth just touching, and put your chin forward without effort as much as you can. Remain in this position for a few seconds. You will become aware of the contraction of the back muscles of the neck. Let your chin be drawn back until the tension in the back of the neck is gone. Note that pushing the chin forward coincides with a break of the breathing rhythm, and that while the chin is held tensely forward you also hold your breath. Now draw your chin toward your throat along the sternum. Wait a few seconds, and note the tension under your chin. Move the chin forward until this tension is gone. Your head is now nearer the correct relationship to the cervical vertebrae than before. Repeat the same procedure all over again with even less tension than before. The neutral position of the head becomes unmistakenly

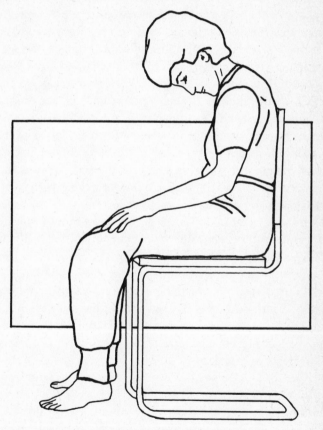

Draw your chin towards your throat along the sternum. (Observation of self while sitting in chair with lumbars slumped.)

clear; that is, you have learned to inhibit the muscular tensions of voluntary origin and to detect finer deviations from the tonic state of the muscles holding the head in this position.

Now, without making any change in the way you are holding your head, push the lowest part of your abdomen forward as gently as you can. If you cannot do so, put your fingertips at the lowest point of the abdomen on either side of it just above the pubic hair and push the fingertips down using only the abdominal muscles to do this; if the rest of the trunk is not tensed and the head is held freely as before, the abdominal push expels air from the lungs. Hold the abdomen forward for a few seconds, and then let that tension go. Still leaning with the lumbar spine against the chair, draw your abdomen in, again as gently as before. If you have not introduced any contractions in the rest of the body, the drawing in of the abdomen equally expels air from the lungs. This is a very important point to notice, as many half-truths are taught about diaphragmatic breathing that make coordinated action quite impossible. Another point of paramount importance must be noted. If you proceed alternating the pushing forward and drawing in of the lower abdomen, you find yourself expelling air at each alternation for as long as you continue doing so. You apparently need never breathe in. That is in fact so—you never need breathing in to involve any voluntary action on your part. If you do not introduce voluntary contractions of the muscles of the neck, throat, tongue, trunk, and diaphragm, air fills the lungs immediately when the expelling effect of the forward push or inward pull of the lower abdomen is over. As the passages of the nose are constricted under the influence of the sharp rise of pressure during such expirations and are free to allow the air in, the inhalation is absolutely inaudible.

Repeat the pushing and drawing of the lower abdomen with the fingertips pressing gently as before, five or six times. If you have introduced no tension that can be voluntarily eliminated (that is, if the neck is in its neutral state and the arms and shoulders lie freely), you will find your breath even and completely inaudible and you will feel a quiet sensation of ease. Note that each inhalation brings a sensation of (1) increased contact surface of the lower ribs with the back of the chair and (2) the opening of the clavicular joints with the sternum. The whole thoracic cage is being lifted while it widens and opens up and is being lowered by the weight of the internal organs and its own weight, thus reducing the internal volume and expelling air.

This sort of breathing accompanies all correct *acture*. Skilled judo masters maintain it even in the heat of intense action, in which case every change of position, which is always initiated in the lower abdomen, expels air from the lungs and replaces it without any conscious attention. Judo masters can thus tire out a dozen young men half their age without any strain. More important than physical prowess is the incompatibility of tonic breathing with the voluntary contractions of the muscles that are produced by habitual fear of failure, doubt, insecurity, and need for approval. In fact, if while learning to recognize the feeling of correct *acture* the student also entertains a motivation parasitic to the one of objective learning, the jaw muscles tense, the teeth are pressed together, the brows contract, the eyes strain, and the lesson does not drive home what it could have. As in all functioning, regulated activity requires continuous feedback between (1) the controlling mechanism and the executive ones and (2) the environment (in this case the body). The improvement of the one adjusts the other to the physical conditions, which in turn improves the first until, if perfection was ever a necessity, the ideal state of functioning is obtained. The material world is what enables the nervous system to form the balance between excitation and inhibition so that a controllable activity of the body can be obtained. The properly adjusted system is capable of completely lifting the inhibition as well as completely damping out the excitation for each function in any plane of activity and enacting only what is considered fitting at the moment. Only when in possession of the full range of functioning on each level or plane of action can we eliminate compulsion to the degree that our action becomes the expression of our spontaneous selves. All creative men and women know spells when they can act in this manner. It is commonly believed that one must wait for the muse or some other inspiration to bring about such happy moments. But mature, creative people have learned to know themselves sufficiently well so that they can bring themselves to the reversible state of *acture*. Thus, they can advertise months in advance the hour when the muse is going to function. This is true of the mature violinist, the mature tightrope walker, the mature male and female in their intimacies, and all those who have learned to differentiate compulsion from spontaneity; they are the only fully potent people.

Stand at the side of a chair. Better put a sheet of paper on it for the sake of preserving domestic peace. Put either hand (let us say, the left) on the back of the chair and your foot that is opposite the hand (in this case, the right) on the chair. Draw your abdomen in flat and try to stand up on the chair. You will find your breath halting and will feel a clear sense of strain in the leg; the sensation of strain persists until something happens in the lower abdomen. Try again, this time putting your lower abdomen in the same state as when the axe changes direction and begins to come down or as in the final state of the sitting attitude. You can now stand up on the chair without any change in breathing and without any sensation of effort.

Having experienced this sensation of fullness of the lower abdomen, you will detect it quite readily every time you change attitude or start or stop any action, provided the action is easy and simple and your breathing rhythm is not broken.

We have used the words *correct* and *right* rather loosely in connection with the abdominal control we have been describing. But there is no *right* or *correct* in itself; we must always ask, "Correct for what?" "Right for what?" The abdominal control in question is potentially correct every time we enact a new attitude or start or stop any action. It is the most appropriate state of the body in which we can switch from one use of ourselves to another. It is, so to speak, the neutral gear of the active body. Whatever else we are going to do, we pass through this state if we are to act in a way that uses our body and mind to the best advantage. The reason for this is that the pelvis is the mechanical basis supporting the body,

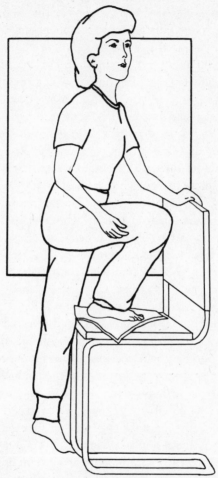

Put either hand on the back of the chair and your
foot that is opposite that hand on the chair.

and it must provide a firm and secure support for the spine. The
mobility of the pelvis is necessary so that the resistance of the
vertebrae to compression is used every time this is possible. This
leaves the muscles free from avoidable impulses that the lower

nervous centers produce in order to preserve the spine from stresses that have a shearing or sliding effect; that is, stresses that are not directed along the spinal curves. The muscles are then free to be directed to our satisfaction without internal contradiction.

This and the fact that the proper pelvic or abdominal control cannot be brought about without balancing excitation and inhibition to achieve unstable equilibrium, until it is possible to enact a projected move, stop it, reverse it, or proceed with its performance at any instance or point in the procedure are the reasons why we call it *control* and why it is so important. When we want to do something and find it difficult, there are always unwanted contractions due to unrecognized motivations that we enact. We must force ourselves to a sufficient level of excitation to overcome not only the objective difficulty but also the internal resistance. Somewhere between the head and the pelvis we enact what corresponds to our personal experience of being weak, of being inferior to the task, of not being good enough—or of trying to appear to be or being the opposite of these—in short, compulsion.

Now, first you must try to get up on the chair in all the ways you can imagine. Afterward, establish the fullness of the lower abdomen so that the whole body can bend forward without the slightest relative change of the head and the whole trunk all along the spine (the bending being performed in the joints of the legs only; that is, in the hips, the knees, and the ankles. Meanwhile, make sure that none of these joints is fixed in space and prevented from moving). It is possible, by moving the pelvis through space so as to continuously compress the spine against the head, to get up on the chair without any sensation of effort, and without any change in breathing. If you are accustomed to acting with great power, you may find no difference in the movement when it is performed one way or the other. But you will soon find a difference if you apply the reversibility test. Try to perform the movement so that at any instant you can reverse the movement of the body without delay or effort or break in the breathing rhythm. This reversibility will become possible when you have learned to act so that the work is being done by the muscles capable of moving the body; that is, by the muscles having one end attached to the pelvis, so that the muscles of the limbs perform only the directing and guiding functions. The fullness of the lower abdomen, which is felt when all parasitic contraction is eliminated, is the best reference by which one can reinstate the correct posture without having to keep in mind the innumerable, detailed, relative alignments of all the body segments. Beware of making will efforts or of trying to grasp a mental picture of correct *acture;* the correct action can only be learned through actual experience.

The importance of lower abdominal control in the sexual act is paramount. Orgasm is an involuntary reflective excitation involving muscular contraction of the entire pelvic floor, including the hips and the abdomen. If freedom of movement is restrained by preexisting contractions, orgasm never fully develops and is most of the time nipped in the bud. Contradictory motivations are sensed as resistance; that is, there is great muscular effort, with stiffness of the neck and shoulders, disorganized breathing, and no gratification that can be sensed.

You will perhaps better appreciate the importance of correct abdominal control if you observe yourself while establishing the sitting position as before. Notice that when you remove your back from the back of the chair and obtain the fullness of the lower abdomen, your anal sphincter relaxes quite distinctly and contracts again as soon as you lose the fullness by retracting the abdomen flat. The anal sphincter contracts in synchronism with the orgasm rhythm, and maintaining it in a state of contraction cannot help but retard and interfere with the normal course of orgasm. Some people contract the anal sphincter deliberately in order to delay the beginning of orgasm. Contraction certainly helps in that respect, but the orgasm that follows is more or less indifferent.

Because the right abdominal control frees the pelvis from unwanted muscular contractions, sets breathing at the personal unhampered rhythm, and consequently relaxes the muscles of the lower jaw, mouth, and hands, it does in fact prepare the body for parasympathetic dominance as much as possible. Thus we achieve what well-coordinated people do spontaneously (with the belief that all people act similarly). And we obtain an advantage over these "normal" people, for they do not know how they succeed and are only all right as long as they do not fail. But by methodical application of the method of control that predisposes the body for correct physiological functioning, we assure ourselves against such mishaps.

The correct abdominal control obtains in every rapid change of attitude that has all the features of proper action described earlier. You can observe it in good golfers when they are swinging a club, in good singers, skaters, dancers, and in every man and woman capable of gratifying sexual intercourse, which includes full orgasm.

In the course of teaching better *acture* and coordination, one is struck by the torturous ways most people arrive at achieving their goal of eliminating certain movements of the pelvis. Both men and women exclude from their *acture* any pelvic attitude that might suggest sexual intercourse or bowel evacuation. When one demonstrates correct movement, one notices that most pupils are clearly conscious of this attitudinal suggestion and some even express that awareness. Many proceed so reluctantly and with such obvious internal resistance that only the example of the teacher and his matter-of-fact attitude encourages the less inhibited pupils, so that by their combined example the others can be brought to follow suit. Once their faces relax and the correct result is obtained, it is pointed out that the corruption of *acture* is always the result of adjustment to the environment, that many possible movements are excluded and that we use only those which are sustained by the environment, so that in fact, the social environment forms the paths of our nervous system. The importance of this teaching lies in that it enables students to lift the inhibition of childish notions of decency and vulgarity, which are ignored by all mature people. One can then convincingly demonstrate that people with mature minds and bodies do use their pelvises quite freely and that nobody finds anything peculiar or indecent in their manner. On the contrary, they are admired for their spontaneous and graceful action.

The occasion is then used to show each individual the connected limitations associated with the exclusion of pelvic freedom. The stiffness of the hip joints, which does not allow the knees to open to the full skeletal limit, for example, depends on the habitual refusal to do so because of emotional inhibition. Such muscles are not short but habitually contracted, and you, like my students, can recover their full range, not by prolonged exercising and stretching, but here and now, by lowering the threshold at which contraction is sensed. First, this is effected, in the usual lying position, by asking the pupil to open the knees as widely as one can do in comfort. Then pressure is applied to force them together, while the pupil is invited to oppose this force by trying to open them. This pressure is maintained for thirty seconds or so until the effect of induction manifests itself, and the contraction of the inner muscles of the thighs relax in reciprocity to the excessive excitation of their antagonists, which are being contracted in the effort to overcome the pressure applied to the knees. The pupil is invited to close his eyes in order to eliminate their control; the only source of information from the limbs that is left now is the kinesthetic sense. The pressure is then gradually decreased and the pupil is required to maintain unchanged (by sensation alone) the state of tension in the inner muscles. When the pupil feels that he has opened his knees to the same limit as they were before, he is invited to open his eyes and convince himself that his muscles have "lengthened" and that his new level of zero contraction is considerably lower than before. With some people, one or two repetitions are sufficient to restore the full skeletal range; others need a few more; and those who only improve partially must be dealt with individually. This is learning in its essence, as the result is obtained by readjustment of the control mechanisms so that the information from the muscles is now better related to reality than before.

Note that the result is not obtained by exercising, repeating, and stretching, which would at the same time exercise the faulty action. Improvement, instead, corresponds only to the difference which the conscious effort of will produces in favor of the focused object. Moreover, stretching means elongating the muscles while they receive impulses that cause contraction; the elongation is obtained thanks to the deformation of the muscle fibers being pulled beyond their elastic limit. Such stretchings produce the familiar pain in the muscles that lasts for several days until the damage is healed, sometimes from seven to fourteen days, depending on age. After that the muscles are as short as before, so that if their normal length is to be maintained one must keep on stretching them in spite of the pain; the healing process is expected to allow for the enforced length of the fibers. However, as everybody knows by experience, it is enough to give up training for a month or so and the whole painful process must be repeated.

On the other hand, the method described allows the restoration of the full range of the muscles by reeducating the central controls and eliminating contradictory impulses. The advantages are quite considerable; the essential quality of muscles is contractibility and not length. The induction method increases the contraction range, and therefore also power. The increased length obtained is accidental; this just happens to be the normal length of a healthy, uninhibited muscle.

The popular toe-touching business is an example of the improper means of remedying one of the widespread limitations on the range of pelvic movement. As long as the cortical inhibition for lengthening is not lifted, the simple mechanical deformation of the muscles must be continuously repeated and life wasted in order to live. People who are very keen on this sort of exercising show through their very keenness their compulsive tendencies in a rationalized way. Uninhibited, spontaneous people, like uninhibited children, can touch their toes without exercising. They use the full range of the pelvis in tying their shoes, soaping their feet, resting in unconventional attitudes, and so forth. They enjoy, beside the futile capacity of touching their toes, the complete mobility of the pelvis as a result of fuller swing of inhibition and excitation control, hence, also fuller emotional swings, fuller sexual orgasms, and fuller social range of friendship.

It is very difficult to convey adequately the idea that abdominal control is a dynamic quality. Most people even when in direct tuition tend to static fixity and often "keep" their abdomens permanently held in what they consider to be the correct position. There is an essential difference between "correct position" and this state in which the body feels like a well-knitted whole, yet weighs less and is more flexible, with the joints as free as in the smoothest, most perfectly oiled mechanism. It must be learned and remembered that we are concerned with *acture,* and not position, with a manner of *doing* and not a manner of fixing oneself even if it is in the most perfectly statuesque position. It must also be remembered that abdominal control is to the body what the keystone is to the arch—you cannot have an arch with a keystone only; the other stones must be as carefully hewn as the keystone. The pelvic region is the foundation of movement, that is, the foundation of life. It bears the genitals and must be free from compulsion and rigidity, and able to move literally in all directions, rotating around the body's center of gravity as a sphere around its center.

The fullness of the abdomen makes the pelvis very nearly a spherical body, the center of which is the center of action. The first sacral vertebra is the point where all stresses in the body cross. This point must be allowed to move freely and is the representative point of the body in all action. In all impotence, mechanical, emotional, sexual, or otherwise, there is compulsive fixity and rigidity in the body which restrains the motility or the gradation of movement of this point and restricts it to exact trajectories, while others are more or less excluded by habitual compulsion. Dissolution of anxiety is subjectively felt as a recovery of a degree of freedom of motion of the center of the pelvis. The tonus of the abdomen is affected by relaxing the eyes, the mouth, the shoulders, the genitals, the anal sphincter, the legs and toes, the fingers, the ribs, and (most of all) the head.

In any particular case of impotence, including sexual impotence and frigidity, there is a lack of motility of the pelvis and defective abdominal tone due to personal experience, as opposed to biological inheritance.

The major problem is the recovery of spontaneity in self-direction and the ability of moving freely from extreme excitation to absolute inhibition on each plane of action. In the body, this expresses itself through the recovery of the full range of all articulations, not only of the major joints but also of the vertebrae, particularly the articulations of the head joint and the pelvis.

Now lie down on your back, extending the head and limbs as effortlessly as you can. Put your hands on your abdomen, with the fingers just touching it. Three points are of special importance: (1) the one point lying about an inch below the navel, and (2 and 3) the two points above the pubis on either side of the abdomen where one can dig in the fingers on both sides of the strong abdominal muscles in the axis of the body. Push the abdomen out so that the first point raises your fingers as high as possible without causing the chest and shoulders to stiffen. Try this a few times until you can fill your lower abdomen without enacting anything else. At first you will not be able to do so. It is enough, however, to direct your attention to inhibiting all the other contractions that you are aware of. Gradually you will become aware of those that you do not sense now.

After a few trials, push the abdomen forward sharply, but without violence and let this movement expel the air from your lungs. Repeat five or six times until you think you can do it well enough. Now put your fingertips at the two lower points in your groin, and push the abdomen forward so as to raise your fingertips with the point below the navel rising equally. The abdomen feels round and blown up like a balloon or a football. Now try to raise the two lower points *without* raising the first one below the navel. You may find it completely beyond your ability; this need not worry you. Try again, paying attention that you do nothing else with yourself above the navel, and pay especial attention to the small of your back. If you manage to push the two lower points forward with the point below the navel raising as high as before, you will feel the small of your back filling out and touching the floor. If you now begin by letting your spine touch the floor from the pelvis to the shoulders without a break, you will find that you have no difficulty at all in pushing the lower two points forward without making any change in the state of tension in the region below the navel. If you continue a few times, you will notice that the abdomen feels as if the balloon is rolling gently toward your face every time the spine touches the floor. If you were expelling air every time you filled your abdomen by pushing it forward, you will now suddenly feel like producing a deep grunt, something like a vowelless "hrrrm" wanting to come out just after the initial flow of air has started. After a few trials, you may now try to push the two lower points forward without the movement of the pelvis which brings the small of the back into contact with the ground. Continue these movements for a few days until you can differentiate between them and produce any one of them unerringly on the first try. You will see for yourself the effect of the refined control of the lower abdomen. It is important to know that you are only learning to use some of your unused controls, and not examining yourself for something you ought to be able to do and cannot. Some people—for example, those who have had the good fortune of being left to grow with neither too much kindness nor too much harshness and who had no premature emotional trials—will be surprised to find that other people need instruction in what is to them so natural and obvious that they never had the slightest suspicion that it may be otherwise. To such people many of the things taught in this book will justly seem like teaching mother to peel potatoes. The only benefit they can derive from the reading is that they will know not to change their ways by imitating admired persons in their manner of doing except perhaps on those planes in which the admired person's action is much better than that of most other people.

Now stand with your feet wide apart, the knees held vertically above the feet. To be more precise, try to create a vertical plane passing through the middle of the patella and through the femur, which would pass also through the tibia and the middle of the heel and would touch the side of the second toe facing the big toe. Both knees should always remain in these vertical planes when standing or moving (unless the opposite intention is the object of the act). When the knees flex to lower the body, they move in their respective planes away from the angle where they would meet were the planes real; in other words, your knees necessarily go further apart when flexed. This is the correct anatomical motion of the knees, in which they can support the body without strain. If the hips have no unnecessary contractions and the lower abdomen is tonically held, the leg hangs correctly from the hip in this fashion.

Now your knees are slightly bent and the hip joints are moved backward as much as possible short of holding the breath and stiffening the shoulders. Fill the lower abdomen by pushing it forward and down so that the lumbar curve is fully formed. Let the chest be kept free of contraction, resting on the firm foundation formed by the pelvis and the rounded, full abdomen, so that the shoulders lie low. Then bring the head up until your nose projects vertically above the lower abdomen. The head can be brought to right alignment by bending it back on its articulation on the atlas until the back of the cranium is stopped by the muscles of the neck. Open your mouth, and let your tongue out to touch the chin. (This is possible if the lower jaw is fully let down and forward and the throat is freed from tension, with the breathing left to itself.) With the tongue out as described, free your neck from tension and let the head tilt forward. If no alteration of the configuration of the lower jaw and tongue has taken place, the head will stop in the alignment in which it is when the body is tonically held. The head should be left alone and free without doing anything else besides relaxing the neck muscles that were used to bend it back, not by actively doing anything to lift it. The less effort involved in the whole procedure, the nearer to the correct result you will be. Your nose will now be more or less vertically positioned above your lower abdomen (the previous test being more reliable than the position of your nose, the length and form of which were not taken into account).

Put your hands under your lower abdomen and lift the whole mass by rotating the full abdomen until you can, simply by shifting the eyes downward, see the third finger after the index. This rolling of your abdominal mass upward should expel air from the lungs, while rolling it downward to the original position should equally expel air. If the alternation of the upward and downward

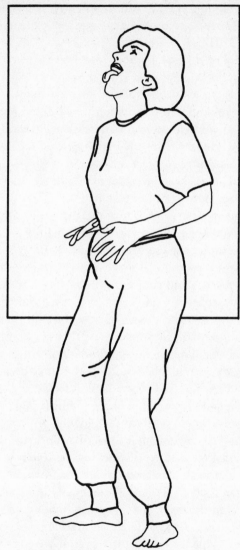

Open your mouth and let your tongue
out to touch your chin.

rolling of the abdomen is performed properly (that is, without any contractions of the chest, shoulders, and neck and at intervals of a few seconds from one another), you will find it difficult to become aware of the instant when you breathe in, as this is now performed automatically, as it should be.

Repeat this breathing out about a dozen times. Then try to perform the rolling of the abdomen upward and letting it drop down without the help of your hands. Remember the movement is of little use unless the rest of the body is perfectly motionless. When all unnecessary contractions are removed and the rolling of the abdomen upward can be performed without strain and exhaling, repeat it about twenty times or so.

The next step, after a rest, is to resume the original position and to roll the abdomen upward without the help of your hands.

Hold it in the extreme upward position for thirty seconds or so, letting the breath continue, through allowing the chest to do what it will. A few trials will suffice.

After some proficiency and ease have been acquired, the rolling upward of the full and round abdomen should be performed against the opposition of your hands; that is, the hands should push the abdomen down while you roll it upward. If your control skill is not good enough and you tense the arms, neck, and shoulders while doing the two contradictory acts, it is better to tie a wide piece of cloth (something like a cummerbund) fairly tightly around your waist and perform the blowing of your lower abdomen (to round it) and rolling it upward against the opposition of the tight cloth. Provided the instructions are followed exactly, the tone of the abdominal wall will rapidly improve. In a few weeks (under personal supervision, in considerably less time than that), a marked improvement of the bouyancy of your whole body and in the countenance of your face will take place.

You may be able to feel the difference at once in the following exercise. Get a chair and stand in front of it as if ready to sit down; then stand as just described and adjust the frame as before until the spine is vertical from the sacrum to the atlas, which results from the just-described adjustments. Then fill and round the

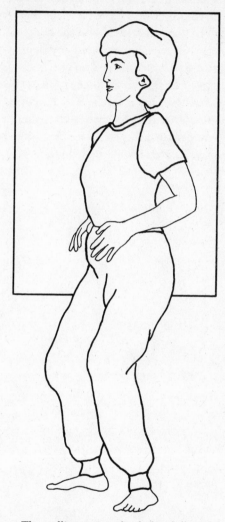

The rolling upward of the full and round abdomen should be performed against the opposition of your hands (while standing).

lower abdomen, lift it with your hands as before, and sit down slowly, lowering the body by bending the knees and letting your pelvis down onto the chair. I say you *may* feel the difference, but your posture may be good in general, and the body will be lowered as one whole piece, just as usual, without any halting of breath or unnecessary strain; if so, you will find no difference. On the other hand, you may have bad posture and—in spite of this description —you may still have so much strain that it will be some time before you benefit sufficiently to even become aware of the improvement. (With personal supervision, the difference may be made so obvious as to appear as a revelation.)

18. A Little Philosophy

Now that you have some rudiments of control for shifting excitation from the sympathetic to the parasympathetic dominance, you should be able to bring yourself to the neutral state in which the fullness of the lower abdomen is present. The body stands more erect, breath becomes even, the muscles clenching the lower jaw begin to release it, the mouth muscles relax, and the head can follow the eyes in all directions without any preparatory change of position of the neck and shoulder joints. The body and mind are rigged to enact any clear motivation. The somewhat loosened knot of tangled motivations can, therefore, be further examined and manipulated until we can find the end of the thread that matters.

Our object is to discover what it is that you really want. It is not an easy task at all, and you certainly do not know it yourself. Had you known it, there would always have been a sufficiently dominant motivation enabling you to use yourself to that effect. And if that had been the case, then this book would reveal to you nothing that you did not already take for granted, and that was also, although perhaps vaguely, obvious to you.

The most difficult cross motivations to recognize are the self-assertive ones, mixed up with the recuperative ones. This is in fact the most pernicious complaint of our age in general. On the social level, this is the age-old unsolved conflict between society and the individual, namely, collectivism and individualism. We are at the same time the most important person in the world (the world that counts for us, that is), and of utter insignificance, from a universal point of view. What does it matter to the world of yesterday, or to the world of a few years from now, whether we can see, walk, or think? Yet how great is our disappointment that we cannot do something as well as other people can? Some of the best human brains have dwelled on this conflict for a long time, and periodically one or the other mode has prevailed. Complete humility and utter insignificance has been taught by the great religious teachers, and mad self-assertion is espoused by their opponents.

There is no solution to this problem, because when we ask the question we inadvertently prepare a frame into which the answer must fit. We expect and we believe that truth is exclusive, unique, and absolute; that a fact is unqualifiably so; and we look for a unique and definite answer—whereas in reality we cannot find a single example of such definiteness even in the simplest particle of matter. An electron appears as matter at the instant that we can recognize it, and as a wave in other circumstances. The greater the randomness of a phenomenon, the more precise and predictable is the law that is based on it. Truth, fact, certainty, probability, significance, and anything else are valid only in a given domain and inapplicable outside that domain, and may be both or neither on the border line. Within the boundary of our body and in a restricted space and period of time around it, we are the most important part of the universe, but outside these limits we are of no importance or significance whatsoever. We are masters in the precincts of our immediate selves and slaves outside of them. But neither of these assertions is of any practical value unless we accept the state of affairs as it is.

Recognizing our insignificance, the unimportance of what we think, do, or cannot do, we find ourselves in full mastery of ourselves to the potential limit of our ability. That sort of unstable equilibrium that is abandoned in each action and recovered for the next is the essence of human maturity. To achieve that mastery within the limits of ourselves, we must sort out the motivations that originate from physiological tensions of our bodies and those that are grafted onto them by habits formed under the duress of dependence. Once we can recognize what we enact, we begin to feel in control of the situation and can preserve our peace of mind in spite of adversity. Some concrete examples will make this point clearer.

From the sitting position, with the abdomen properly held and without changing the position of your feet, try to stand up. First try to lift yourself straight off the chair. You will feel your breath halting and the abdominal muscles tensing; you will have lost the right control. Try again; lean your body forward on the chair without any change in position of the spine except leaning it forward. Proceed by moving the lower abdomen forward first a little, and try to stand up. You will again feel your breath halting and the quadriceps of your thighs (the big muscles above the knees) contracting powerfully; your breathing shows strain and your movement is incorrect, because your abdomen is improperly controlled. It has lost some of its fullness and become stiff. Finally let the full abdomen move forward, leading, as it were, the body to the point where you find yourself on your feet without any change of contraction of the abdomen. This time your breath is not interfered with at all. There is no feeling of effort, and the contraction of the quadriceps is hardly noticeable.

Correct abdominal control is normal to all children before some patterns of motion have been excluded from their normal usage by the inculcation of arbitrary and erroneous ideas of caution, prudence, or decent and indecent movements. Once the forgotten control is reinstated (and everybody can recall the time of early adolescence when they frequently enjoyed it), the readjustment to the new behavior is comparatively easy. One then feels able to generalize the attitude that one knows in all spontaneous correct action when it happens. Musicians, dancers, and in general people who use muscular skill as a means of expression would find their apprenticeship considerably shortened and the level of skill to which they can aspire heightened by a methodical use of lower abdominal control. Unfortunately we cannot proceed here with elaborating the whole course of methodical training. If you have succeeded in getting the feel of it, you need not worry—progress will be slow, but continuous.

CROSS MOTIVATION

One of the most pernicious motivations that persists unrecognized in many of us is the longing for approval. This is often encountered in people who have grown up in homes where kindness is instilled with an absolutism and severity amounting to despotism. Such parents consider themselves as the elite and bring up the child to feel that she is unique, that her refinement and delicacy are unmatched. Such a child is goaded to excessive politeness, cleanliness, and goodness by continuous appraisal of even the intention to obey. Necessarily she is rebuked and ostracized for any tendency in the other direction. The child finds herself constantly submitted to a parental scotch shower of affection and rejection that distorts her emotional balance. She gains approval from her parents when she denounces her little friends because they do not behave as her own parents want her to behave. While she thus gains parental affection, she loses the ability to form friendships, a loss that she will suffer forever afterward.

Affection and appraisal do not become compulsive if the child is fortunate enough to have a sensible teacher during the schooling period. Otherwise the need for approval becomes so intense that the child will often denounce herself and even confess invented misbehavior in order to elicit from her parents or teachers approval for her uprightness. The pattern becomes so ingrained that the person keeps on finding fault and reprimanding herself, to the point of really hating her wicked self. All spontaneity is thus rooted out, and the person has an inner eye opened constantly, watching, torturing, and punishing herself. People like that are afraid of stammerers, people with tics, and the word *impotence.* They have at some time or another admitted their wickedness, weakness, cowardice, or impotence, because they could not live up to the absolute standards that were mirrored before them by compulsively upright parents. Having admitted their failings, they keep on expecting their deserved punishment—which rarely comes, unless circumstances develop unfavorably and the compulsive habit becomes really obsessive. To the casual observer such people may even seem very gifted, as they have spells of feverish activity and real growth during which they have a fair chance of improving their *acture.* Very often, however, they seem to find the upward slope too steep and find themselves in a corner —one quite reasonable by common standards—but which is to them a tangible proof of their failure and inadequacy. In general, all this self-criticism is out of touch with reality. They are just as potent as anybody else and not worse than anybody else. It is only that with them the habitual compulsive need for approval makes their self-assertive urges too intense and unremitting. Their musculature tenses, and they can never let themselves go completely; hence their sensation of failure of sexual power, which is never measured by the emotional quality of the relationship, but only by the number of acts and their duration.

Mr. K. L. is a good example. He is married, has three children, and makes a comfortable income. To all outside appearances he is a happy man. But his sexual life is absolute misery. With a few memorable exceptions, erection fails him just when he wants it, and very often halfway through intercourse. He has never had sexual relations with a woman other than his wife. He had psychoanalytic treatment for several years, which helped him a great deal in general, but this complaint persists. He suffers less than before, but has periods of great depression and has intercourse only once every few months. He waits for a special state of mind, which is difficult to obtain because of impaired digestion and heartburn. He suspects a stomach ulcer or perhaps a cancer.

Mr. K. L. is extremely polite, immaculately dressed, and very tidy, rigid in his demeanor, stomach drawn in, chest immobile and breathing shallow, lower jaw clenched, and mouth tightly contracted.

His face, carriage, and general demeanor are those of a man demanding both recognition and the acknowledgment that he is a very nice man. Now, obviously it is a good thing to be a nice man, or to alter one's behavior so as to be nicer than one might otherwise be. But it is another matter entirely to have a compulsive need to be nice. In a society in which we depend on each other as completely as we do, it is necessary to be nice to each other, but not for the sake of obtaining approval from all around us. It must be remembered that we are not directly concerned here with morals, the appropriateness of action or its purpose, but with the ability to enact what is wanted or the inability to do so. Had there been no compulsiveness in Mr. K. L.'s behavior, and had he been capable of enacting what he wanted when he thought it expedient and capable of refraining from doing so in other cases, the whole question would be beyond our scope. His movements and carriage showed that he was compelled to conduct himself in that manner primarily in order to obtain confirmation and approval, without which he felt his emotional security to be compromised. His behavior indicated action corresponding to unrecognized motivation, so that each act carried with it a habitual parasitic element. As in all cases where no dominant motivation is possible because of compulsive background motivation, his action lacked reversibility where the question of approval was involved. Therefore, his action could not fit reality. He could not stop himself from enacting his unrecognized motivation all the time even when circumstances demanded the exact opposite. He was nice whether he wanted to be or not, in spite of himself and even in spite of his better judgment.

To many people, this may seem to be an ideal state of affairs—perhaps even too good to be true. So such behavior was bound to be strongly sustained by the environment. Everybody, himself included, approved of his behavior, and the attitude and habit was thus formed. Two important points should be noticed: First, his unqualified nice behavior would in the long run not only be expected but also demanded from him as a due. Moreover, any inconvenience or resistance he encountered as a result or a consequence of his habitual and compulsory behavior was, in fact, due to a positive action produced by him.

Of necessity, he was enacting a number of other unwanted acts that he could not recognize because the level of background excitation was constantly too high for detecting weaker ones. As a concrete example of his habitual attitude, it was suggested to him that his penis at that moment was contracted and shrunk, the blood vessels constricted, and erection not only inconceivable, but even difficult to visualize.

He admitted that was so, but could not see any connection. This suggestion was ventured without any visual or other evidence for it. His general attitude, face muscles, drawn-in lower abdomen, and chest held rigidly in a state of inspiration all showed that he was enacting conflicting motivations. One behavior showed that he excited his self-assertiveness and expected to compel my approval of his demeanor, while the other showed doubt and anxiety. Muscular tension and interrupted, uneven, and shallow breathing go together with vasoconstriction and are evidence of the inhibited state of the antagonistic parasympathetic vasodilatory influence—so it was safe to venture the suggestion made.

There was little doubt that he maintained this habitual attitude all the time, even when approaching his wife. That is, his frame of mind when he approached her was one of expecting approval and recognition of his kindness and general superiority, although he was inwardly convinced of his inadequacy. He was, therefore, constantly on the lookout for the slightest indications of approval to confirm him in his intention. If they were not clearly forthcoming, the slightest and most insignificant detail would discourage him. In this specific state he cannot bear delay, because his erection starts and falters following the movements of self-assertiveness. In this case, there is no real sexual tension to be relieved; instead, a tangled mixture of self-assertive motivations has grown up. The self-assertiveness is so intense and the sexual urge so inhibited by it that he is often glad to meet with frank disapproval, as this justifies him (in his own eyes) in giving up his intention and thus brings his inner struggle to an end. As soon as this happens the inhibition is lifted and he has a full erection, whereupon he feels confirmed that he is not at fault and approves of his own behavior. A feeling of ease and restfulness pervades him. He falls asleep fully erect. Thus, as soon as he stops seeking approval or when giving it to himself, he is fully potent.

He is unable to understand that in fact he is absolutely selfish and not nice at all, because he is not in the least concerned with his wife's attitude at the moment. The whole problem presents itself to him as being only a question of his perfection, and virility and whether or not he acts kindly. He has not the urge for friendliness that sexual tension creates. There is only the dominant need for approval, cross-motivated and mistaken for sexual desire. This is, in fact, the faulty action; he does not approach his wife because he is feeling the sexual tension that impels him to seek intimacy, and the intercourse can only release sexual tension. Selfishness is an essential contradiction in a situation where two persons unite for mutual gratification. He was selfish, because he acted on a self-assertive plane altogether; the physiological significance of the act was entirely compromised. In the best of cases, such an act could only accomplish reproduction (as indeed it did) but must be (as it usually was) a complete failure as far as full gratification goes, or as concerns the regulation of the recuperative functions vis-à-vis the self-assertive ones.

If someone starts with the habitual attitude of searching for approval—that is, a self-assertive motivation that makes vasodilation difficult if not impossible—then his entire frame is fitted for anything except intercourse. In these circumstances, he has to compel himself to produce an erection and thereby create some sort of sexual tension. He produces that erection by a will effort, which in fact consists most probably in (1) contracting the anal sphincter and the diaphragm or some other part of the abdominal region, and (2) visualizing a personal intellectual picture of erotic hue.

During the learning process, K. L. often complained that he could not think of anything, that his mind was blank. The mind becomes blank when two conflicting motivations of equal intensity are presented at the same time. The old habitual mode of acting is still acceptable, because it cannot be completely inhibited before another pattern of action is substituted. When we feel like discarding a habitual pattern, the only one that has ever been enacted for a given motivation, and before the new pattern has been produced by the body, it feels strange. We feel as if we have lost the power of control over our body, or the power to think. If no positive step is taken to provide a new and better pattern of action at this stage of complete readiness to discard the old one, the old pattern will be reestablished and reverted to before very long. If the use of the old pattern is made physically impossible, it will continue to be visualized in the imagination as long as no new pattern has been sensed at least once in the body. To understand that the new mode of action is better is not enough; one must feel it to be better through the physical experience of the body.

The reader knows the rudiments of the technique of bringing the body into a state from which it can be brought to perform any act without further preliminary change. In this state, any change of attitude or action will expel air from the lungs freely and without any conscious attention. From this state the reversal of the habitual pattern becomes possible. But before reversing the pattern one should first become proficient at inhibiting it. When the idea of intercourse presents itself in the usual way, the lower abdomen should be brought into the state of fullness already experienced, breathing made even and rhythmic, and the idea of intercourse completely rejected (that is, one must decide not to enact it). The abdominal control can then be further improved, breath made simpler and deeper, and muscular tension in the hip joints, the shoulders, and the neck as well as in the anal sphincter and around the mouth made to lessen even more. That state maintains itself through the pleasant feeling it engenders. If sexual tension reappears, it should be rejected once more in the same way as before. The dialogue that follows is presented without the pretense of being verbatim.

But what will my wife say if I behave in this peculiar manner? The approval pattern was so deeply rooted in Mr. K. L. that it could be found in practically every act or thought he had. He was advised to recall that his wife often refuses his caresses. Yet nothing terrible happens to her nor to him; her manner does not seem queer to him, and, likewise, nothing terrible will happen if he does as advised. Moreover, she cannot know at all what he is doing, as the entire process is internal and nothing can be observed outwardly that differs from ordinary behavior. Once the rejection of the old pattern is mastered, one becomes aware of a wealth of faults that one can normally not detect at all.

You said something about a crop of faults I am going to discover; well, I now think that there is nothing I can do really properly. I have been thinking about my wife simply saying, "Leave me alone," when she does not want me. And the terrible effort I have to make even to think of doing the same thing revealed to me so many faults in my behavior that I am at a loss to find what is the most significant one. When I first felt reversibility in the lesson on sitting up, I thought I knew what it meant. In the last few days I have felt on several occasions something very similar but in my soul, not in my body. I have succeeded in rejecting the idea of intercourse, and to my surprise I found that I had an erection, but without any feeling of sexual tension at all. I did not know when it started, and became aware of it only when it was complete. I wanted to have intercourse, but my wife's attitude brought me back to my usual mood, and all was over before I could do anything. What I am trying to say is that perhaps it is not my fault at all. I dare not think about it, but I feel that perhaps with another woman I would not have the difficulties I have.

It is premature to think of any major changes in your life at the moment, before we have unearthed the sexual motivation from underneath the heap of other extraneous and parasitic ones. My contention is that, with the anatomical and neurological apparatus being intact, as in your case, it is enough to learn not to interfere with the lower centers of the nervous system to obtain their proper functioning. As long as we can point out improper *acture* and control, it is futile to take any steps that you might regret later when your behavior is adjusted to reality. For the moment, you must admit that you do not know what is happening even in your own body under your own directives and that you cannot judge what is beyond your potential ability. Sexual relations cannot be adjusted by one person alone, and your wife has certainly as much to learn as yourself. But at this stage, relations with another woman would be more than a handicap to you. You have certainly thought of other women before, and something else besides the moral deterrent stopped you from establishing sexual relations outside your home. So long as you are driven to intercourse primarily and compulsively by self-assertive motives and not by spontaneous sexual urges toward a person, your anxiety will probably be even more acutely sensed and your difficulties greater than usual with another woman. The need for approval would not be reduced by just any other woman, but only by one who would not evoke it. Had you had the luck of coming across one at the right time, the whole course of your development would have been different. On the other hand, you could hardly have done other than you did, for your *acture* was such that you would have rejected such a woman. The need for approval made you seek out your wife who sustained that need and satisfied it in such a way that you felt safe with her. If you look for another woman at this stage, you are almost certain to pick one who has the same tendencies as your wife. At the moment, your anxiety is also lessened by the amount of blame you can put on your wife. Thus, from every point of view you must wait for some time yet before you are in a position to make a decision on such an important matter.

If you look back on your behavior now that you have gained some proficiency in reversibility, you must admit that you are far from being the nice man you paraded yourself as. You were certainly not a very kind husband, and not a very easy one. Indeed, you were faithful only by compulsion, and likewise, your wife cannot be judged on her past behavior. Undoubtedly she needs some learning too, for she is now adjusted to your past self, but this is not the moment to take any drastic steps. As you realize yourself, your sexual function is perfectly sound; your trouble is in your social adjustment. You maintain a childish need for approval. When you gain complete reversibility and are able to isolate the sexual motivation and act on it, you will be in a position to make decisions. You may find your attitude becoming that of a man to a woman and not that of an adolescent who wants to show how strong he is or how well he has learned to do his homework. This change will help your wife to become a mating companion as well as the legal companion and mother of your children she is now.

I am completely disoriented. I realize that my troubles are of my own doings, but what am I to do?

Your question is the best sign of improvement. Maturity means taking responsibility for one's existence in every respect. Your quest for what to do and not asking to be helped is a healthy tendency. But nobody can tell you what to do except to be "good," "pull yourself together," or give you other directions that you cannot comply with. You know very well what you would like to be; the question is to learn to do it. If you could enact what you want, your problem would be solved as far as you are concerned. You still have incomplete extension of the hips, tension in the muscles of the inner thighs, and your chin still tends forward. Your posture shows that anxiety is not completely resolved and that you are not yet completely successful in projecting a clear body image and mobilizing yourself on one dominant motivation. The muscular pattern of the old *acture* in the cortex presents therefore centers of inhibition and excitation that distort any new projected thought or direction into that habitual way that you came to dislike. It is this muscular tension that reinstates the whole situation. You produce the contraction of the muscles of the pelvic region, and especially of the anal floor, with the idea of supporting and maintaining the erection. These contractions are linked in your previous experience with fear and doubt, and you feel you have to proceed with intercourse while it is feasible. You cannot but be a nuisance to your wife, who cannot possibly become sexually inclined at a moment's notice, while you yourself have been toying with the idea for some time. Thus, you are not impelled by sexual urge, but by the need for approval of your virility, and you create the sexual situation for another motive. Therefore, the problem of failure is the central point in your body image. You probably proceed compulsively, without feeling any friendliness toward your wife, only familiarity. You express no tenderness nor virility and do nothing to tune your wife in to the situation.

I know that. I read long ago that one has to caress, kiss, and otherwise fumble other parts before penetration. I have been trying, but I find it awkward, and my wife does not like it either. I begin to understand why.

These explanations may be different from the insight you have gained through previous analytic experience, but they are in essence only another more concrete way of indicating "mother complex." They relieve some of the anxiety, but to make any real difference it is necessary to learn the correct way of projecting orders to oneself and have the frame in a state fit to enact them. We have learned to inhibit action when it is to be corrected or altered; you should try to transfer the learning onto more important things for you. When you are about to act in your usual way, halt yourself and give up the idea altogether. Let the erection subside; it is not the last time you will have one and you need not exploit the opportunity. If it is the last, so much the better for you, then you need not learn anything and you are free to attend to your daily business without trouble. All virile men often find more important things to do and do not take advantage of each erection. You have thus obtained rough reversibility, which needs further improvement. Go on refusing penetration until you can kiss, embrace, cuddle, and caress solely for the fun of doing so, continually inhibiting the idea of penetration and refusing to allow the erection to manifest itself. The self-assertive motivation being inhibited, the fear of failure and the anxiety linked with it will be inhibited too. By reducing all tension in the abdomen, pelvis, neck, mouth, eyes, and allowing the body to breath, parasympathetic excitation or dominance will be invited; you will find delicate pleasure in kissing, caressing, and courting. In fact you will be going through the course of apprenticeship that most people went through in their adolescence (when the idea of penetration was inhibited by moral compulsion). You will, by the way, stop being the gloomy and high-strung bore that you were in your past sexual experience. Paradoxical though it may seem, by acting solely for your own pleasure you will gratify both your wife and yourself.

I am sure that if I keep on watching myself, none of the things you mentioned will happen.

As during our training, you may find some initial difficulties. They disappear with increased skill. You have had that experience and felt the results. You recognize the sensation that helped you during the lessons; try then to learn from your own body, in your own language, what no understanding will do for you. We do not want to succeed once and always be at the mercy of losing the ability. This is what is meant by the full range of a function. If you learn to act correctly while you watch yourself, you may find it difficult in the initial stages; but you cannot act without clearly projecting orders to your executive organs, and, as in all learning, there is a stage of exaggerated conscious control. You will gradually get rid of it, and you will not know how you have learned it, any more than you know how you learned to write or count. You spent years on learning these things; it will take you a ridiculously short time in comparison to learn by learning correctly.

I have had a very hectic time with ups and downs, happiness and despair. I have done as you last told me, and even though I inhibited the idea of intercourse the erection did not disappear entirely. The penis remained full and felt weighty. It did not shrink as it usually does, but there was no urge for action. I felt a peaceful warmth all over my body. My wife complained of her usual headache, which always irritates me. For a while I felt my mood changing, but I succeeded in retaining the warm feeling. Then the devil pushed me, and I found myself telling my wife all about my seeing you. I couldn't imagine myself doing so before, because of my discreetness, and I was rather proud of myself for being able to do so. I expected her to be glad of my confession, because she always complains of my keeping things to myself and keeping her out of my inner life.

But I did not know what was coming to me. My wife completely lost control of herself, and a terrible stream of invectives poured out of her. I was the most selfish brute, nice and kind to everybody except her; I had not the slightest consideration for her feelings, trampling her in the mud. How could I be so coarse as to discuss her sexual behavior with a stranger, expose the last corner of her privacy without giving even a thought to her feelings about the matter? She cried and sobbed, passing from self-pity to deep hatred toward me. At last, exhausted, she fell on the bed with her face downward, apparently calm except for frequent convulsions of her whole body.

I did not know what to do or say. I was afraid to interfere with the queer and strange sensations in myself. It grew on me that I did tell her everything, as a child would tell his mother about a nasty thing he had done. I knew that I did it expecting her to be happy about my confession and to relieve myself of my secret. I felt she was right about my selfishness and the lack of consideration for her feelings. Indeed, I never thought of her at all. For the first time I really saw how distorted my conduct is by this cursed longing for approval. But I was calm; I felt sorry for her, but not guilty. I went near the bed, knelt, put my hand on her shoulders and told her I was sorry; I really was. I never was so sincerely sorry.

I did not care about being so unmanly and went on telling her how much I suffered from my incapacity. That I did not do it for my own sake only, but that I wanted her to have what she would have had if she had married another man. I lay on the bed near her, and she put her head on my chest. I felt her completely relax, my hand stroked her hair. I became aware of a full erection, but without the usual tenseness in the body. I felt my face relax and did not dare to move for fear of spoiling it all. I refused myself intercourse, but the warm feeling continued and the fullness in the penis persisted though there was no more erection.

We went to bed with the feeling of sincere intimacy. I was erect again and I penetrated, but I felt no desire to move and remained motionless for some time, but continually fully erect. I felt some contractions in my wife, and I lost my semen without ever making any movement at all, yet I think my wife was gratified.

There is no limit to perfection, and there is more to do before you reach faultless performance. But we must follow our rule, that is, ask what we can do now. The first thing to do is to consolidate the acquired improvement, then to generalize it. Next time you bring yourself to the state you have just experienced, inhibit the new pattern and reinstate the old one again. You improve the reversibility of both patterns and the contrast between them increases, so that you feel better in the new state than you otherwise would. This will help to inhibit the old pattern for good. You will also get rid of your apprehension of its fortuitous reinstatement.

If you try to remember, you will find that during the days of using yourself in the new way you did not suffer from your habitual digestive troubles. You must continue to maintain this rate of improvement, which helps you to maintain the new control and your health in general.

Now that you have consolidated your position, and you are

more sure of being able to bring yourself into the right state of mind and body to enact the wanted motivation, we may continue the disentanglement of the approval pattern from sex. If you examine all that you told me, and especially the way in which you told it, you will find that you have been motivated by the urge to obtain approval from me more than you recognize. You had to tell me what you did, but the manner of telling betrayed your expectation of my recognition of how nicely you behaved and how good a pupil you are. But you do not remember now the teacher who taught you to read and do simple fractions. Without him, you would not be able to be what you are, yet he is of no importance to you today. You owe him nothing except a debt of reverence, and that more by convention than in reality. You owe me nothing, and I hope you will learn your lesson as well as you have learned your reading and arithmetic. I will join your other teachers in the corner of oblivion in your memory. The mature person does things for the sake of doing them or because they are expedient, and not for the sake of approval by his seniors, equals, or subordinates.

With respect to your wife, the approval motivation is still too pronounced. You say you "did not mind being unmanly," you "did things for her sake," and so forth. Nothing is wrong in these attitudes in themselves, but in your case they are of the greatest importance. You may continue to do them again because they are expedient or because you like doing them, but they must not enact themselves unrecognized. Habitual patterns have a tendency to reinstate themselves with any element of the whole being enacted. If you leave in a number of the old habits, you will find, in the long run, the entire pattern reinstated, and come to believe that there must be after all something really wrong with your inheritance. Whereas you can see and feel now that the question is entirely one of knowing what and how to do.

You often speak of doing "as other people do." If such comparisons really mean anything to you, we may consider our goal achieved, because a considerable part of our society is satisfied with a sexual life far below the level you have reached now. Some further progress will come in due course, as your behavior now will probably produce quite a different response from your wife. She will not need headaches so often to avoid having sex with you. You often betrayed your conviction that she really had no desire for intercourse, and indeed she had nothing pleasurable to look for.

We could bring about an added improvement by teaching your wife the management of motivation and correct action. She submitted herself to you, but did not seek to release any body tension. Security and sex are intricately entangled in her. Secretly she probably thinks that she is no good for you, that had you married another woman with greater "sex appeal" you would be a happier man. It is a comfort to her to think that you are lustful and selfishly seeking pleasure. At the same time, your caresses only irritate her, because she feels herself being acted on as an instrument. Indeed, she is right; you said yourself that you used caresses mechanically, for the purpose of sex and not because you like doing so.

I suggest that for some time you go on using your better mode of doing and proceed to unravel your self-assertive motivations from the others. With the reduction of muscular tension and anxiety you have achieved, and with further improvement of reversibility, you will feel even smaller differences than before and therefore you will feel something wrong before acting very improperly. You will be cultivating self-reliance and assuming responsibility for all the resistance you encounter. Your aim is to establish a balance between the assertive, protective, and recuperative functions and to learn to control this balance and shift one way or the other as circumstances demand. You cannot achieve such mastery without a sufficiently dominant motivation allowing full involuntary orgasm with intense gratification. Even in the need for approval you must achieve reversibility and learn to care for approval but without compulsion.

As soon as you allow any parasitic motivation to become as important as this one, you will find yourself in difficulty again. Extraneous motivations of social, moral, and self-assertive origin cannot be entirely eliminated in our society, and we are bound to enact some of them by habit. We must, however, not allow them to become dominant, in which case we feel powerless. We enact something by long-standing habit and cannot recognize ourselves in the act, and thus we are forced to believe that some evil spirit has taken possession of us.

In case of difficulty, remember that your mind cannot act at all by itself; it needs a body, which you have to learn to control. And remember that the mind is formed by our personal experience. Bring your body and mind to the appropriate neutral state by the means of which you now have the secret. This unstable state is to be abandoned only for definite action and resumed afterward in readiness for the next; one action for self-assertive functions and another for recuperative ones.

Bring your body into the state of fullness of the lower abdomen and fullness of the penis, as you have learned to do, and anxiety will fade away. You will be able then to enact what is expedient and the sexual motivation will become important only when the body tension will demand it. In the past, the sexual motivation pressed itself into the foreground most of the time, because it was impossible for you to separate it from the self-assertive use of yourself which is kept active by the environment. The sexual problem had become the problem of your life. It can now be relegated into its proper place. Once the tension is fully released, there is nothing to keep the motivation alive. Both your self-assertive and recuperative functions can now swing higher and deeper, as they do not come together, but come one at a time. Your work, your leisure, and your sex life will deeply interest you and will become more and more intense. You will *live,* instead of vegetating as in the past.

PREMATURE EJACULATION

Mr. P. X. is a pleasant young man, solidly built. His neck is stiff and strong, his head is held forward with the chin protruding, his pelvis is hyperextended. His feet are rather turned with the toes outward. His manner is pleasant, but self-conscious. He clears his throat repeatedly in the first few minutes and uses his handkerchief to dry his face for no apparent reason. He has a kind but rather meek look in his eyes.

Closer inspection reveals flat transversal arches with toes slightly hammered and all touching each other. There is no space between the big toes and the other toes. The heels are slightly turned outward. The chest is bulky and practically motionless in the position of inspiration, and his breathing is mainly due to the lower ribs moving laterally.

He is rather pale, somewhat short-sighted. He holds his upper lip immobile, never uncovering his upper teeth. He is periodically slightly constipated, with his feces gradually becoming reduced in volume until he has no feces for one day at all, and then the cycle starts anew.

Mr. P. X. is serious minded and not given to jokes and fun. He is extremely methodical and painstaking, a hard worker, and he indulges in self-criticism.

He stands stiffening his legs and buttocks and uses strength in all his movements, but lacks swing and ease. In rotation, he gets terribly contracted and stiffens all his muscles, leans forward, and does not let himself go. He holds his breath and holds his pelvis as if withdrawing his genitals from a threatening gesture. His knees turn inward, and all the faults of his standing become exaggerated.

This young man is very secretive about intimate body functions and succeeds in telling very little of relevance when he does try, using all kinds of abstract words without finding the word that is obviously on the tip of his tongue. He is single and has a number of intimate friendships with different women. He complains of disappointingly brief sexual acts, especially in the beginning of a new relationship. He has almost invariably a mild bilious attack after repeated intercourse and feels stiffness in all his body for the next day or two, especially in the region of the lumbar spine. Sporadically, everything is simpler and easier; he can control the onset of orgasm, and the aftereffects are less marked than usual. At such times he feels poised, light, stands taller, and does not stiffen his body. He does not know exactly how it happens that he suddenly finds himself in that special state in which he feels he is really himself. But he knows that something normally prevents him from putting himself in that frame of mind. His feeling is as if he is normally following a groove from which he cannot deviate, and that in his bright moments he feels that he somehow manages not to engage himself in this groove. Once he succeeds in avoiding the initial slippery path into the groove, he feels that he has, so to speak, free will and is really master of the situation.

He also resents his lack of firmness with other people; without premeditation he is quite incapable of telling anybody off even when he knows that he ought to. He puts himself in the other person's shoes and imagines how it would upset the person, and he cannot muster up the courage to inflict the suffering he imagines he would cause. At the moment he finds it easier to suffer himself, but later cannot forgive himself for his weakness.

In his adolescence he was unable to address even a family gathering, let alone a public meeting, though he often felt he had some pertinent remarks to make. Even now, when caught unaware he cannot stand up for himself, although the following instant he knows the very excellent retort he should have made. Sometimes he is much better in this respect, especially when in that happy frame of mind referred to before. But somehow in this state the situation he would like to tackle rarely arises.

Reeducation of this intelligent and pleasant person moved rapidly. He was sure that he was a normal person and secretly believed himself exceptionally gifted, which he undoubtably was. Yet at the same time he believed himself suffering from some mental kink, but he also found that most people were in the same position. He would have never consulted a psychiatrist; the idea seemed preposterous to him. But he was keen on physical education and was eager to learn to control his body.

I had no difficulty in obtaining his agreement that his reaction to quick movement was to stiffen himself, which resulted in his wide stance. I showed him that when he was standing with his feet wide apart, not only was he more stable but at the same time he was also incapable of changing position without first shifting his weight onto one leg or lowering his body. He could see that he could only resist the change of position by stiffening and trying to preserve his balance. How did he come by this stance? Could it be corrected? What could he do to change it? And what does it have to do with premature ejaculation?

A wide stance is an infantile feature. Until the lumbar curve is formed all children stand wide. The pelvis gradually becomes mobile and extension of the hip joints complete. In a properly matured body, the pelvis participates in every movement and oscillates rhythmically in every step. A long apprenticeship is necessary before the complete mobility of the pelvis is reached. There must be sufficient cause to prevent the person from reaching the normal state of mature pelvic control. It may be congenital deformity, accidental injury, or a complicated arrested learning process. Obviously, the preferred immature lower mode of use must have a peculiar personal attraction to the individual and fulfill a sufficiently important need, and it must also be sufficiently recurrent to prevent any further development.

Usually a single event of great emotional intensity is the origin of arrested learning, but unless the event is strong enough to cause irreparable harm, normal development will be resumed sooner or later. To perpetuate arrested learning, a long series of situations that evoke the initial incident must recur; that is, the symptom must be sustained by the environment in order to become one. And, as already noted, imagining a punishment that cannot be reality-tested fulfills all the requirements for conditioning a response that later may seem to have come out of the blue.

I have also pointed out earlier the importance of observing facts as they are. Thus, we stand wide to prevent falling. So a person standing wider than necessary without an anatomical reason for doing so is avoiding falling, whether he knows it or not. The habit must have been formed through the fear of falling initially and continues to be sustained by a feeling of insecurity that somehow the environment evokes in him recurringly.

Children are often prematurely encouraged to stand; from time to time they fall heavily on their seats with a disagreeable jerk of the head. Adults are in the habit of shouting loudly, with the intention of giving the child confidence or making him forget the misadventure. But loud shouts only make the child jump, blink, and contract his body. There is no harm in all this, but parents will continue this game for their own enjoyment or to show off to their friends; they often succeed in distorting the attitude of the child to approval and linking the idea of the ridicule with pain. The danger is in the general overemotive attitude of parents who subject a child to appraisal and reproval much too often and too intensely. The child learns to avoid the disagreeable experience by preserving the mode of standing he has mastered and in which he feels safe and is now reluctant to try new attitudes, so the normal course of learning is temporarily arrested. If left alone, he will soon pick up the normal course of development. However, future reversion to the old manner is made much easier now. Circumstances and events of quite an ordinary or indifferent character, that have no special effect on other children, may cause this one to revert to the old manner, which feels safer and more pleasurable.

In the case of P. X., an older brother delighted in pushing him back onto his seat with increased violence every time he could do so without being found out. The younger brother, who could not yet move properly to avoid falling, found that stiffening and leaning forward was a remedy and soon learned to get ready at his brother's approach. In this state of compromised security, all happenings acquired a special significance that they did not have before. If his elder brother were patted before him, he imagined his parents joining hands with his brother. They were all so strong, and they loved each other! He was constantly on the lookout, and therefore saw things where there was nothing to see.

Once people become aware of a new pattern they can see it everywhere. When immature minds realize something with a certain intensity, they then continue to see it where it is and where it is not. When the Struggle for Existence, the Red Menace, and the Trust Conspiracy are suddenly realized in a state of compromised security, they continue to be found everywhere, all the time.

In our subject the idea of the need to be ready was evoked continuously all through his waking life. However, in fact, he is never ready, as he has never formed an adult erect carriage with complete extension of his neck and back, the only attitude from which any movement is possible without preliminary getting ready. He felt he was doing right (1) by increasing his static stability, (2) by selecting from among the great variety of events only those where his posture assisted him to find the sense of safety, and (3) with the same consistency, by carefully avoiding all those events that involved parting with the preselected pattern. The vicious circle started in an environment that produced it and continues to maintain it. It cannot stop, and the pattern becomes habitual. He now avoids games and acts that demand swift, spontaneous responses such as hopping, jumping, and in general all acts involving complete and correct hip extension.

All his relations with the outside world are thus formed around an infantile mode of behavior based on a faulty notion that static stability and strength are the proper means to employ in all cases. In the preselected conditions, in which all situations where these means are useless or inoperative are avoided, the infantile behavior is consistently satisfactory. Indeed, he can even find ground for congratulating himself on his rocklike stability and solidity and his ability to foresee and get ready for all events for which sufficient warning and time to get ready are available, as he believes that this will enable him to cultivate strength and get his own back on his more agile and mobile friends. Unfortunately for him, the proper functioning of the human frame is incompatible with continuous rocklike immobility. The human frame is essentially an unstable structure fitted for continuous change, and it functions smoothly and at its best only when maintained in a state that makes all attitudes equally realizable.

When we have relieved all the unnecessary tensions (that have been built up in the course of development as the only means of reacting to the environment available at that time, that have become useless at present), we can obtain a better and easier comportment. Thus, if we eliminate from standing all that is extraneous to it, such as standing *manly, femininely, authoritatively, nicely, efficiently, arrogantly, proudly,* or *meekly* and all the other cross motivations that we cultivate in childhood and adolescence with such wholehearted conviction of doing right, there remains standing as dictated by the structure of the body and its nervous mechanisms. A stance that is rare, but of which we are all capable.

Because body experience is necessary in order to form the paths in the motor cortex of the brain, people erroneously think that to work hard repeating an action—exercising ad infinitum—is necessary before they can do what they both wish to do and feel they cannot. The only reason the whole erroneous idea could have become so widespread is because of this one element of truth in it. To take a simple example, if for some reason we decide to learn to stand on the head using the method of exercising (trying to do so) we soon find that we do not have enough willpower to persevere, because when we first begin, we never succeed in standing for any length of time. The proper way to learn to do things is to learn how to learn first. Fortunately, this is not the only procedure yielding results, but it is the only one that increases the capacity to learn and not simply to improve in this or that detail, with every new act presenting new difficulties and a new spell of interminable exercising.

Behavior in general—the behavior of the well-adjusted as well as that of the ill-adjusted person—must be considered as a dynamic phenomenon. There is considerable theoretical advantage in so viewing it. All behaviors are "a priori" each one as good as the other, but in particular conditions one is more expedient and becomes the normal behavior, while the others become neurotic. This point of view is particularly helpful in our times, when different social orders compete with one another and well-adjusted people find themselves suddenly incapable of integrating themselves into the new conditions and even prefer to die rather than deciding to change their habitual patterns.